THE
STUBBORN
FAT FIX

THE
STUBBORN
FAT FIX

EAT RIGHT TO LOSE WEIGHT AND CURE METABOLIC BURNOUT WITHOUT HUNGER OR EXERCISE

KEITH BERKOWITZ, MD
AND VALERIE BERKOWITZ, MS, RD
WITH ALISA BOWMAN

Foreword by Mark Hyman, MD, author of *Ultrametabolism*

RODALE®

© 2009 by Keith Berkowitz, MD, and Valerie Berkowitz, RD

Photographs © 2009 by Rodale Inc.

Rodale books may be purchased for business or promotional use or for special sales. For information, please write to:

Special Markets Department, Rodale Inc., 733 Third Avenue, New York, NY 10017

Printed in the United States of America

Rodale Inc. makes every effort to use acid-free ∞, recycled paper ♻.

Photographs © Thomas MacDonald/Rodale Images

Book design by Christina Gaugler

Library of Congress Cataloging-in-Publication Data

Berkowitz, Keith.
    The stubborn fat fix : eat right to lose weight and cure metabolic burnout without hunger or exercise / Keith Berkowitz and Valerie Berkowitz.
       p.   cm.
    Includes bibliographical references and index.
    ISBN-13 978–1–59486–828–3 hardcover
    ISBN-10 1–59486–828–X hardcover
    1. Reducing diets Popular works.   2. Metabolism—Popular works.   3. Dietary supplements—Popular works.   I. Berkowitz, Valerie.   II. Title.
    RM222.2.B4535   2009
    613.2'5—dc22
                                          2009002284

Distributed to the trade by Macmillan

2 4 6 8 10 9 7 5 3 1 hardcover

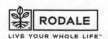

RODALE
LIVE YOUR WHOLE LIFE™

We inspire and enable people to improve their lives and the world around them
For more of our products visit **rodalestore.com** or call 800-848-4735

Contents

Foreword

We are disoriented, dazed, and confused by an abundance of misinformation, contradictory nutritional claims, and lack of clear, practical steps to address our personal and our global struggle with excess weight. On our planet, more people are now overweight than are starving. Obesity has exceeded malnutrition as the number one cause of death worldwide, resulting in 29 million deaths from preventable lifestyle disease such as heart disease, diabetes, cancer, and dementia.

Solutions to this crisis are not immediately evident because our national food policy is controlled by an agriculture and food industry that profits from increased consumption of "fake foods" or "Frankenfoods." Yet buried within that mountain of misinformation and deliberate deception, the science of what to eat, how to create health, and how to automatically restore normal metabolism and self-regulate our weight, is screaming to be known.

Now Dr. Keith and Valerie Berkowitz clear up the misinformation. From their personal and professional experience and from the overwhelming scientific literature, they present the wisdom of practical, responsible clinicians who have successfully helped thousands of patients lose weight for good.

The Stubborn Fat Fix's brilliance lies in its simplicity and accessibility for everyone. Eat more real food. Move a little, rest a little, and add metabolism-boosting nutrients. That's it. But the implications for this are broad and profound. What's more important than what we *don't* eat is what we *do* eat.

It is no mystery why we are sick and fat. With each of us on average consuming 66 pounds of high fructose corn syrup, 158 pounds of total sugar, mountains of trans fats, and more than 3,500 chemicals (MSG, aspartame, and food dye, to name a few) added to our food—as well as a gallon each of toxic pesticides every year—it is a wonder we are walking around at all.

Real food is something most of us rarely consume—whole foods just as they are found in nature—a whole fresh vegetable, not salty canned versions; a whole brown rice grain, not processed flour; a whole fruit, not fruit juice; a whole nut instead of trans fat and sugar-laden processed nut butters; and beans, seeds, lean animal protein such as fish, chicken and eggs. Think farmer's field, not food chemist's lab.

If you do this, then counting fat grams, calories, and carbs is unnecessary. You can eat more and weigh less.

All of the obstacles to weight loss disappear when we put foods that we are designed to thrive on in our bodies and limit artificial additives that block, interfere, or alter our normal appetite and metabolism. You will no longer suffer cravings, hunger, or deprivation. This book is about possibility—the possibility of effortless weight loss by focusing on health first.

The Stubborn Fat Fix is a bright spot in the darkness of an obesity epidemic that should be read for its common sense, science-based, simple, and extraordinarily practical road map. This map will not only create sustained and mostly effortless weight loss, but radically transform your health and well-being at the same time. And here's the simple reason. The same things that make you sick make you fat. And the same things that make you fat make you sick. So when you eat real, fresh, whole foods and take care of your body's basic needs for movement, rest, relaxation, and nutrients, not only do the pounds fall away, but diseases disappear as well. So the side effect of *The Stubborn Fat Fix* is preventing, reversing, and often curing chronic illness. Not bad.

Mark Hyman, MD
December 2008
Author of UltraMetabolism: The Simple Plan for Automatic Weight
Loss, *and* The UltraMind Solution: Fixing Your Broken Brain by
Healing Your Body First

Acknowledgments

We are extremely thankful for the opportunity to help you improve the quality of your life. Thanks to Rodale Inc. for helping us spread the message that eating healthy isn't just about losing weight but about getting well and living longer, too.

Specifically, we'd like to thank Adam Campbell at *Men's Health*® magazine. You've been a great supporter and friend. Also, our editors, Kathy LeSage and Andrea Au Levitt: Thank you for discovering us, believing in us, and encouraging us every step of the way. This book would never have happened if it weren't for you.

Jeremy Katz, our agent, has been a mastermind who not only coordinated this winning team but even lent some of his personal recipes to the cause. Alisa Bowman spent many tireless hours writing this magnificent book, developing recipes, and managing our deadlines. Thanks to Dr. Mark Hyman for contributing the Foreword.

To the Goldstein and Berkowitz families: It was your solid base that allowed us to explore this alternative way of eating and wellness. To our three children: You give us daily inspiration and always make sure we are on course.

A huge thanks also goes to our clients, especially those who allowed us to tell their stories within the pages of this book.

Beata Moniuszko and Binni Ipcar: You are the heart and soul behind our practice. You each play a critical role in the success of our patients at the Center for Balanced Health.

We also thank the late Dr. Robert C. Atkins. He was and still is an inspiration to us in changing the way we practice medicine and nutrition. He was a pioneer in this field.

THE
STUBBORN
FAT FIX

THE OVERSPENT BODY

We wrote this book for the multitudes of people whose physicians have told them to lose weight "or else."

Or else you'll need blood pressure, blood sugar, or blood cholesterol medication.

Or else you'll need bypass surgery.

Or else your diabetes will result in blindness, amputated limbs, or organ failure.

Or else you'll die.

Or else. We don't use those words in our practice. We don't because we understand that you have been trying for many years to lose weight. We believe you. We also know all too well just how many physicians, friends, and spouses have already said those words. We know that the words *or else* do not motivate people to lose weight.

You don't need to hear these words because you already know them. Michael certainly did. When he came to our practice for the first time, he was more than 20 pounds overweight, diabetic, and terrorized by "or else." "In the past six years, I've gone from doctor to doctor," he told us. "Each one prescribed me a different batch of drugs, none of which worked." By the time Michael came to us, he was taking $400 worth of prescription medications every single month, was fed up with doctors, and was terrified. "I'm afraid that I'm going to die," he said.

He wanted to see his children grow up, attend college, get married, and have children of their own. He desperately wanted to lose weight. What was stopping him? His body was bankrupt, and his physicians were trying to pull him out of that bankruptcy by getting him to stress his body even more—more in the way of exercise, more in the way of effort, more in the way of fear. Sure, various physicians had suggested he eat less. They hadn't, however, shown him how to eat less in the midst of everyday crises such as hunger, cravings, and fatigue.

Once we outlined our nutritional and supplement plan and gave Michael the tools he needed to stick to it, Michael started losing easily. His blood sugar evened out. Without the peaks and valleys in blood sugar, his cravings diminished. His hunger transformed into satisfaction. His energy levels normalized. His metabolism improved. He cut his monthly drug bill by 75 percent. He regained his confidence, and his life. Oh, and he also lost 20 pounds. You can read the details of how Michael did it on page 8, and we'll offer more stories of patients who lost anywhere from 10 to 70 pounds just by following our simple, sustainable plan. Keep reading to find out how you can get the same great results.

WEIGHT LOSS THAT WORKS

Over the years, we've helped hundreds of people just like Michael. We enable weight loss by encouraging our patients to do something that at first seems extremely counterintuitive: Eat more. Move less. That's right. Eat more. Move less.

Of course, you've heard you should do the opposite. You hear it all the time: eat less, move more, right? Yet this may be the worst advice to follow, because cutting back on food while ratcheting up your exercise can trigger sudden drops in blood sugar that increase cravings, decrease energy, and leave you hungrier than ever. This either gets you nowhere or gets you even heavier than you were before. These are your body's cries for help. There is an underlying cause of your hunger, preoccupation with food, and lack of energy.

On this program, by eating more and moving less, you will recharge your metabolism so you can finally, once and for all, lose weight.

You'll do it without the deprivation associated with most diets, too. We don't expect 100 percent adherence to our plan—in fact, we "build in" opportunities to indulge. We've included luxuries such as ice cream, chocolate, and a glass of wine with dinner. You'll be able to enjoy the foods you love, and keep right on losing. More important, we'll show you how to have these foods without suffering extreme spikes and valleys in blood sugar. You'll learn how to eat to bring your body into balance.

A LITTLE ABOUT US

In 1999, we met Dr. Robert Atkins, tried his diet, and lost 20 pounds. Of course, we'd read the news stories and heard the experts claiming that the diet raised the risk for heart disease, so we made sure to monitor our health with regular blood work. You know what? Neither of us experienced a rise in blood cholesterol, blood pressure, or blood sugar. That experience won us over to the merits of low-carb diets and was the primary reason we signed on to work at the Atkins Center for Complementary Medicine. We believed Dr. Atkin's approach was truly revolutionary.

We eventually went out on our own, founding our private practice, the Center for Balanced Health in Manhattan. We set about creating a plan that would enable the most resistant body to shed fat *in the real world.* We wanted people to reap all of the dramatic weight loss of lower-carb, higher-protein, higher-fat diets, sure. But we also wanted to make sure they got enough other important nutrients—most critically, the fiber and wholesome foods such as fruits and vegetables that they *weren't* getting before. We also wanted to bring their bodies into balance. We wanted to find a more moderate approach that most people could stick with long term. While we worked and tinkered and fine-tuned, we stumbled onto perhaps the biggest secret to our success.

What was it, you ask?

We devised a way for people to continue to indulge in their favorite high-carbohydrate foods and still lose weight. When most people diet, they temporarily stop buying and eating foods such as ice cream, chocolate, bread, and fruit. Yet you can only deny yourself such delicious foods for so long. When you forgo all of your favorite high-carbohydrate foods, you end up wanting them all the more—and eventually you find yourself *eating* them all the more. Despite withstanding lots of deprivation, you end up overeating anyway, and gaining weight rather than losing. How frustrating! We knew that deprivation was the Achilles' heel of every low-carb plan, so we built in safety valves. No longer would a low-carb diet equal a no-fun lifestyle. No more all-or-nothing, if-I-touch-a-carb-it's-all-over deprivation. We'd created a successful, healthful, delicious diet plan that works long term—even in real life.

By following the program in this book, you'll lose up to 10 pounds in the first 2 weeks and up to 10 pounds a month after that until you reach your goal. You can succeed. You can lose weight. Read on to find out how.

THE NO-HUNGER DIET PLAN

To allow you to lose weight without hunger, we use an individualized five-pronged approach that includes:

A whole foods diet: Based on your health, weight, and eating habits, you'll choose from two eating plans that vary in their amounts of recommended carbohydrate foods. These eating plans feature whole

Shannon Bryant **Lost 50 Pounds!**

I've always struggled with my weight. My sisters are twigs. The biggest one is a size 4. My mom is a size 6. And then there is me. People assume that fat people eat 500 gallons of food a day, but that's not true with me. I've never eaten huge quantities of food. I'm not a snacker, but whatever I eat makes me gain weight.

In college, my freshman 15 was more like the freshman 40. And my weight has slowly and constantly crept up ever since. I've tried so many diets. I'd lose some weight, but I just could not stick with any of them long term, so I gained it back. In 1995, I went on a liquid diet and lost 50 pounds. I weighed 130 for 2 whole weeks! I was really cute. Then the leftovers from a banquet were stored in my office. I hadn't had a bite of solid food in 4 months. I was working late, and I decided to have some brie on a cracker. It was as if that first bite opened the floodgates of the Hoover Dam. I gained more than 100 pounds in a matter of months. My all-time high was 262.

With this approach, I've lost more than 50 pounds in 7 months and I'm still losing. This is the first diet I've been able to stick with long term. I think it works because it's not as restrictive as diets I've tried in the past. Of course I miss cer-

foods (fruits, vegetables, whole grains, meat, fish, eggs, and cheese) that are free of weight-gain-promoting additives such as added sugar, high-fructose corn syrup, refined flour, trans fats, and refined soy.

You'll slowly add in more carbs as your body allows. You will not, however, have to eliminate your favorite whole foods forever. We include healthful, fiber-rich carbohydrate foods such as avocados, nuts, berries, and olives early in the plan. Yes, low-carbohydrate eating does not have to equal no-carbohydrate eating!

The food lover's pressure valve: You'll prevent that do-or-die moment—when low-carb dieters usually start fantasizing about belly flops into heaping plates of pasta—with regular servings of indulgence foods. These treats do away with deprivation altogether. You can enjoy regular small servings of dessert (yes, you heard right, we're talking chocolate and other sweet treats), fruit, and yes, even bread(!), and still lose weight. A *lot* of weight. We'll show you how, and we'll show you how to get and stay in control, too.

Supplements that heal your metabolism: You'll couple your whole foods diet and regular cheats with a supplement plan specially tailored to your individual body chemistry. These supplements have

tain foods, such as corn and potatoes, but I also get to eat foods that are fulfilling and tasty. For instance, I can eat sea scallops with drawn butter and steak with béarnaise sauce. I am, of course, eating more vegetables—especially celery and cucumbers—than I ever have before. But it's the savory, flavorful foods that keep me on track.

I get stuck more often now that I've lost and regained weight so many times. The plateaus are frustrating. I need a lot of patience to get through them. Not long ago, for instance, I didn't lose an ounce in 4 weeks. To help me get through this most recent plateau, the Berkowitzes suggested something that at first seemed counterintuitive. They suggested I cut back on exercise. I had been weight training three times a week, doing yoga twice a week, tennis once a week, and the elliptical trainer nearly every day. Now I alternate weights with cardio, and I take more days off. The scale is moving in the right direction again, and I'm at my lowest weight in 20 years.

You really do have to be ready to make a life change. You hear all the time that you can't go on a diet. It has to be a lifestyle. That's the God's honest truth. You can't adopt something that is intolerable and think you'll be able to do it for a few months until you lose the weight. You'll never make it. You need to do something that is reasonable, that you can do for the rest of your life. This is that diet.

been shown to balance hormones, reduce cravings, dampen down appetite, and increase your energy and sense of well-being. They'll help restore your metabolism and greatly enhance your weight loss results.

Rest and relaxation: Lack of sleep and high amounts of stress burn out your body. They bring hormones out of balance and increase appetite, both of which cause you to gain weight. We'll show you a simple yet effective plan for reining in stress and improving sleep, so you can reboot your body's healthy hormonal balance and lose weight without hunger or cravings.

The right amount of movement at the right time: On this plan, you exercise only once you feel ready. For many people, that's only after losing a considerable amount of weight. Trying to force your body through intense cardio or weight lifting routines from the very beginning of a diet usually backfires. Why? In the beginning, with your metabolism out of balance, exercise just causes even more imbalance by keeping you in a burned-out state. It taxes your body at a time when you need rest. Plus, you feel tired. Who wants to exercise when they're tired? It's much better to change your eating first and then slowly add in exercise once you feel more energetic.

Most important, we'll support you every step of the way. Based on the hundreds of patients we've counseled over the years, we have a pretty good idea of the varied challenges, excuses, and roadblocks that stand between your current body size and your ideal weight. We'll show you what to eat to reduce nighttime cravings for sweets. We'll help you deal with interference from family and friends. We'll talk you through eating out, holidays, and vacations. We'll help you overcome emotional eating, stress eating, and mindless overeating. We'll even help you break addictions to sugar, caffeine, and starch, dependencies that make weight loss all but impossible.

We're here for you. We are because we've been there. We've not only helped people lose weight, but we've also done it ourselves.

Successful weight loss is about food, of course. But it's also about your spouse, your kids, your friends, your hobbies, your career, and your sleep habits. It's about how often you watch TV, and even about *what* you watch. It's about how long you sit in front of the computer each day. It's about preservatives and additives lurking in your food. It's about your mind-set, and about whether you are a perfectionist or a more easygoing person. It's about what you can live without, and what you can't. Successful weight loss is about hunger and about cravings. It's about learning how to deal with both, and finding ways to overcome them.

Throughout the pages of this book, we're going to teach you about success. First and foremost, we're going to help you become successful biologically. Our diet and low-stress lifestyle plan will help you balance a complex set of appetite signals that trigger you to eat, overeat, and gain weight. Have you suspected that an overactive hunger switch or sluggish metabolism may be the cause of your weight problem? You're probably right.

Second, we're going to help you become successful psychologically. Have you tried low-carb diets before only to fall off the program when cravings for crunchy, sweet, or savory foods overpowered your ability to say no? We'll help you deal with those cravings by allowing indulgences early in the plan and by showing you how to stay in control when you have them. Unlike other low-carb diets that deny you anything remotely resembling a treat for weeks upon weeks, our plan recognizes that some people—many people—simply need a hint of sweetness to get them through some rough patches in the early days. Once you're past the initial phase, you can choose to indulge in ice cream, salty snacks, chocolate, wine or beer, and even bread—so you'll be able to have the foods you love when you want them most. These appetite-suppressing, satisfaction-promoting options will help you stay on track without feeling deprived.

Third, we're going to help you become successful socially. Your family and friends play a huge role in your ability to stick with your dietary approach. You'll learn what to do about the family member who suggests that late-night ice cream run—and how to put those indulgences on *your* schedule, not his. You'll learn how to handle the coworker who tempts you with her candy jar—so you can choose the higher quality chocolate that *really* satisfies.

That's what makes this plan different from others you may have tried. We give you the tools you need to make your dietary changes last a lifetime. We help you fire up your motivation and commitment from day one, and we stick with you every day of your weight-loss journey, offering solutions for common problems you will likely face along the way. We help you understand why your body fights against every single dietary change, and we enable you to circumvent your body and, at times, your mind so you can be successful. Once you lose all the weight you want, we make sure the results of your hard efforts last.

BETTER HEALTH, BETTER WELL-BEING

We'll help you not only drop pounds but also do it in a way that restores total body health and well-being. Throughout this book, you will read the amazing stories of patient after patient who overcame extremely high cholesterol, blood pressure, and blood sugar. We've seen patients halve or even stop taking medications for blood pressure, asthma, and many other diseases and disorders. That's how much healthier they got with our nutritional, supplement, and stress-reducing plans.

Thanks to the wealth of nutrient-rich whole foods and health-promoting supplements, you can expect to see the following health benefits, some of which may take effect within days of starting the plan:

- Sleeping all night long, whereas now you may wake frequently
- Relief of gas and bloating
- Improved mood

Michael Sachs **Lost 20 Pounds!**

When I started this program, I was 52 years old and had been diabetic for 6 years. At 6 foot 4 inches and 230 pounds, I knew I was overweight. I knew I ate too much, too. If I had pizza, I didn't just have two slices. I had six. If I was eating spaghetti, I didn't have one bowl. I had three. If it was sandwiches, I'd have two of them, not one.

Many physicians had told me to lose weight, but none offered me the specific advice or answers I needed to make it happen. I went from doctor to doctor, each prescribing me a new batch of medications, none of which worked. As time passed, my blood sugar rose. One physician even asked me not to return to his practice after the medications he prescribed failed to rein in my blood glucose! He blamed my poor health on me.

By the time I visited the Center for Balanced Health, I was afraid I was going to die. I wanted to be around for my kids, but it didn't seem as if I could get my eating or my blood sugar under control. Dr. Berkowitz sat with me for hours, answering all of my questions. He was compassionate and soothing. He was confident that he could help me. I believed in him and felt comforted by him. I was willing to try anything he suggested.

- Increased energy
- Improved overall health
- Improved blood cholesterol levels and blood pressure
- Improved endurance during exercise

Your sex life will also perk up and joint pain will disappear. You'll also be happier and more confident.

Let's talk about some basic physiology. It will help you understand why past diets have not worked and why ours will.

Our stomach, intestines, fat cells, and organs are all linked to our brains through a complex set of appetite signals, and this appetite system is designed to encourage us to gain weight at every opportunity. Why? Our bodies are designed for famine. Not many hundreds of years ago, we humans could survive only if our bodies encouraged us to eat at every opportunity and to eat more than we needed at any given moment. We survived only if our bodies directed us to rest at every resting opportunity, and to move only when the movement helped us to eat or stay out of danger.

Because of this survival system, we feel hungry whenever we see,

The nutrition plan recommended was logical. All of the meals suggested were normal, whole foods with an emphasis on fiber. I took out most of the starchy carbs, including the potatoes, pasta, and pizza. I limited my consumption of fruit. I started eating five or six small meals a day rather than three huge meals. I snacked on walnuts and almonds. At night, when I had the urge for something sweet, I tried ricotta cheese mixed with cinnamon, sweetened with a little vanilla and stevia. It tasted like ice cream.

It was effective. In 6 months, I not only lost 20 pounds but also reduced my fasting blood sugar by 150 points. I was able to reduce my monthly outlay on medications from roughly $400 a month to less than $100. My cholesterol and blood pressure dropped, too.

I now sleep through the night. When I wake in the morning, I feel rested.

I feel better and look better. As the weight dropped and as my energy levels improved, so did my confidence and attitude. I felt so much better that I was able to apply for and get my dream job of working for a large corporation in the technology field. I now have the problem of needing an entire wardrobe's worth of new suits. Life is good.

hear, smell, or think about food. We can blame this overactive hunger response on a hormone called ghrelin. This hunger hormone, produced in the intestine, rises at mealtimes, when you see food, when you smell food, when you think about food, or when you see food on TV. Ghrelin is what makes your stomach feel empty. It travels to the brain and says, "Feed me."

When ghrelin rises, it's hard to talk yourself through the hunger you feel. You may have just eaten. It may not be rational that you feel hungry, but you do. So you eat.

Food hits your stomach and intestines. As the stomach fills out and expands, nerves register the sensation of being stretched and send the brain the "I'm full" signal. Other chemicals, including a hormone called leptin that is released from your fat cells, confirm this message, telling the brain, "We're really full now." They also tell the stomach to stop sending food into the backlogged intestine and tell the pancreas to make insulin to shuttle blood sugar into cells. The problem is that these signals are sluggish and they don't travel quickly. It takes 10 to 20 minutes for these signals to reach the brain with the "I'm uncomfortably full" message, and, for most people, that's too late. The sluggish response allows us to wolf down much more food than our bodies need at any given time, especially if we are eating quickly.

Depending on what we've just eaten and how quickly the food moves through the intestines, these fullness signals can be fleeting. Once they tell the brain "I'm full," fullness signals dissipate, which is why we're all capable of feeling hungry within minutes after eating large amounts of food, especially if we have an ice cream sundae sitting in front of us.

As soon as you gain just a little bit of weight or throw the system off with too much stress or too much of the wrong types of foods, these messages from the various hunger and fullness hormones get distorted. The hunger hormones grow stronger and the fullness hormones grow weaker. Leptin and insulin levels remain chronically high, and the brain stops listening to them. Instead, appetite signals keep getting through, and you continue to feel hungry, even when you shouldn't. According to the signals that are getting through to your brain, you are "starving," and we mean that literally. Even though you are actually gaining weight, your brain is getting the message that you are wasting away, so it directs your stomach to rumble at every opportunity. You're living in times of plenty, but your brain thinks you're in the middle of the Great Depression.

Muscle cells stop responding to insulin, so insulin has no choice but to usher calories into fat cells. This survival system worked well for us when our next huge meal might be days or weeks away. It doesn't help us out so much today, however, when our next meal is as close as the refrigerator.

BUT I EAT ALMOST NOTHING!

You've struggled to lose weight because your metabolism is not in balance. What is your metabolism? In the simplest terms, it's how the body converts food into energy. Ideally, you want your metabolism to operate much like Warren Buffet's bank account. You want the deposits (what you eat) to balance the withdrawals (what you burn) so that you maintain a healthy weight. This is *not* how most people's metabolisms work. Most people run really fast for a while, and then they run really slow. They put in too many deposits and then spend, spend, and spend. They create highs and lows that stress and run down key body organs and hormones, including:

The pancreas. As your stomach and intestines break down the food you eat into fuel that can be absorbed into the bloodstream, the pancreas pumps out insulin, a hormone that helps your body either store extra calories (as fat) or burn them for energy. Think of it as a master key that opens many doors (cell membranes) throughout your body. Some of these doors are on muscle cells. When insulin fits into the locks on these cells, blood sugar enters and is either incinerated to make energy or stored (in the form of glycogen) for later use. Insulin can also open doors on your fat cells. When it fits into a fat cell's lock, blood sugar is converted into fat and stored in the cell. Some insulin is good—it helps the food you eat go where it belongs. Too much insulin—which generally comes from eating too much of the wrong types of food—is not.

Elevated insulin is the underlying cause of weight gain, unstable blood sugar, low blood sugar, mood swings, low energy levels, and many health conditions such as diabetes, heart disease, high blood pressure, some cancers, and, in women, polycystic ovarian syndrome (a condition characterized by weight gain, infertility, and excess body hair). Elevated insulin is also to blame for metabolic syndrome, an increasingly common condition characterized by three or more of the following factors: abdominal obesity, elevated triglyceride levels, low HDL cholesterol, elevated blood pressure, and elevated fasting glucose levels. When insulin rises and stays elevated, it keeps you feeling hungry, and it stores excess carbohydrates, especially refined sugars, as body fat. As fat cells get larger, they require still more insulin to metabolize nutrients, which leads to even more fat storage and further weight gain. The more carbohydrates you consume, the higher insulin levels rise. This is why high-carbohydrate, low-fat diets actually provide the raw materials for weight gain.

The adrenal glands. These triangular glands sit on top of your kidneys. They make stress hormones (cortisol and adrenaline) and sex hormones (testosterone, estrogen, and progesterone). Daily stress triggers your adrenals to overproduce the hormone cortisol. By getting too little sleep, overworking yourself, or overexercising, you can eventually fatigue them and lose your ability to make the cortisol your body needs. When cortisol production falls, intense cardio can initiate the breakdown of protein stores, leading to a loss of muscle mass and an increase in fat mass. This is why exercise may not always be good for weight loss. Poor adrenal function also lowers levels of testosterone in men, progesterone in women, and DHEA in both sexes. This leads to weight gain, fatigue, low sex drive, insomnia, infertility (in women), and emotional instability (moodiness).

The thyroid gland. Thyroid hormone helps regulate metabolism,

Anette Muscarella **Lost 40 Pounds**

I've struggled with my weight my entire life. I was never the kind of kid who ate a lot of junk food. When my friends were eating hamburgers, I was eating salads, but I was always really heavy. Mom took me from doctor to doctor for testing, and they all said that nothing was wrong with me, that I should eat healthier. It was so frustrating.

By the time I got to high school, I was 40 pounds overweight and whenever I ate, I felt sick. After dinner, I would not be able to do anything because I felt so sick, uncomfortable, unhappy, and tired. Dinner was the end of my night. I was so unhappy about my weight and how I felt. Mom told me, "I've heard of this doctor who might be able to help you. I'll call him right now if you want me to." I told her to make the call. She got Dr. Berkowitz on the phone.

Seeing Dr. Berkowitz was one of the best things that ever happened to me. He was the first doctor who talked to me in a way that made me feel comfortable. He told me that I deserved to feel healthy and energetic again. He told me that I did not deserve to feel sick all of the time. Those words were so comforting to hear.

My tests revealed that my thyroid was a little slow and that I probably had yeast in my GI tract. He gave me lists of foods to eat and not eat and a list of

energy levels, mood, body temperature, and various bodily organs. If your thyroid is not functioning optimally, you will gain weight easily, resist weight loss, feel cold, become depressed, and suffer from dry skin, thin hair, low sex drive, joint and muscle aches, high cholesterol, and fatigue. The American College of Clinical Endocrinologists estimates that 1 in 10 Americans have an underactive thyroid and that half of them remain undiagnosed.

The sex hormones. You may be low in testosterone (if you are a man) or progesterone (if you are a woman) and high in estrogen for either sex. Fat cells store and secrete estrogen, so as you gain weight, estrogen levels rise, which interferes with testosterone and progesterone levels. Estrogen, like insulin, is a fat-storage hormone. When overly high, it also worsens blood sugar control.

The GI tract. There are more organisms living in your gut than there are cells in your body. Many of these organisms are good guys that synthesize vitamins and fatty acids, neutralize toxins, and make hormones. Others aren't. As they ferment the food you eat, they release toxins that can slow metabolism and make you feel fatigued.

Taking antibiotics, eating meat laced with antibiotics, eating too

supplements to take. Within a week I felt a lot better, and I progressively felt better as time went on. I was losing weight, too, but the weight loss wasn't what made me so happy. It was my health and how good I felt. My entire life was better.

As I was losing weight, my friends would tell me that they couldn't understand how I could give up foods like bread, but once I knew that it was the bread that made me feel bloated and sick, it stopped tasting as good to me. Once I made the connection to how bread, pasta, and other starchy foods affected me, it was a lot easier to not eat them because I felt a lot better when I avoided these foods.

Now that I have lost 40 pounds and improved my GI health, I can have small amounts of those starchy foods, but I know my limits. I have to stick to small portions. This isn't a death sentence. I can still have what I want, in moderation. I know that eating certain foods will make me sick; and if I'm sick, I'm not going to have a good time. I'd rather have a good time than eat unlimited amounts of certain foods.

Now I'm less self-conscious in social situations. I'm more outgoing and able to speak my mind. I enjoy life so much more.

little fiber, or consuming too much sugar can throw off the delicate balance of bacteria and other organisms in your gastrointestinal tract. When antibiotics reduce levels of healthy bacteria or when sugar over-feeds yeast and unhealthy bacteria, levels of healthy bacteria drop and yeast and harmful bacteria proliferate. Yeast secretes toxins that weaken the immune system and cause the following symptoms: gas, diarrhea/constipation, bloating, gastric reflux, post-nasal drip, brain fog, fatigue, increased appetite, headaches, rashes, and food allergies.

Research at Washington School of Medicine in St. Louis shows that an imbalance among the types of bacteria in the intestine can even cause you to absorb more calories from the food you eat. The research-ers found that overweight people tended to have lower levels of a type of intestinal bacteria called *bacteroidetes* and higher levels of another type of bacteria called *firmicutes*. Because the firmicutes bacteria do a better job of breaking down carbohydrates, they cause the body to soak up more calories from carbohydrate foods.

Despite popular belief, yeast overgrowth isn't something that only affects women. Plenty of men have it, too. We recently treated an execu-tive who had been diagnosed with sleep apnea and was using a breathing machine to keep his windpipe open at night. It turned out that a yeast overgrowth in his GI tract was causing an excessive amount of post-nasal drip. Within 4 days of starting our diet, the man was no longer using his breathing machine, and his wife no longer complained of him snoring.

No matter which or how many bodily systems are not working the way they're supposed to, the end result is the same: Your metabolism stops working effectively, too.

WHY EATING LESS DOESN'T WORK

"Weight loss is easy. Just eat less."

Over the years, we must have said that to hundreds of patients, even though only a few were successful. We now know why. This conven-tional advice—eat less, exercise more—only works if your metabolism is in balance. For everyone else, the divide between wanting to eat less and actually managing to do it can be as wide as the Grand Canyon. If your metabolism is out of balance—as it is for 90 percent of the patients we see—calorie cutting and portion control will only make you hungrier, more tired, and eventually fatter.

Here's why. If you reduce calories the way the U.S. government and many medical establishments suggest, you do so mostly by reducing fat. That means you're still consuming most of your calories from carbohydrates. All of the carbohydrates you eat turn into blood glucose, and, right now, your body probably does not handle blood glucose effectively. Until you fix your metabolism, a high-carbohydrate diet will cause blood glucose to quickly rise, which will cause your pancreas to pump out the hormone insulin, which will direct 85 percent of excess glucose into fat cells, causing blood glucose to drop and resulting in hunger, and starting the cycle all over again.

The same is true for exercise. Many physicians cause an endless amount of frustration by continually suggesting that their overweight patients start exercising. They tell you, "Move more and you'll burn more calories and build muscle mass. This will speed your resting metabolic rate and you'll lose weight." As with portion control, it sounds good in theory, but it doesn't always work. You probably don't need us to tell you this. Do you feel like going for a run right now? We didn't think so. Does exercise hurt? We thought so. Are you too tired to even think about moving your body? Yep, sounds familiar.

When your metabolism is not working efficiently, exercise fatigues an already overburdened system. Rather than improving metabolic function, it can often make it worse. In particular, it places a heavy burden on your adrenal glands—glands that are probably already exhausted. You can't fix your metabolism by willing yourself to exercise and praying and hoping that someday you'll be in shape. Rather, you must do the opposite. You must rest and repair. You must sleep, relax, and fix your metabolism with the right diet and supplements. Only once you make your metabolism more efficient can you start and maintain an exercise program.

Don't misunderstand us. We're not telling you not to exercise—ever. We're not saying that exercise is bad. We're only saying that it may be bad for you right now. Right now you need to concentrate your efforts on repairing the problem. Once you bring your metabolism back into balance, exercise *will* accentuate weight loss by bolstering metabolism and burning calories.

We hope you're relieved to know that you do not have a lack of willpower. You don't have a personality defect, either. We hope that you now understand that weight loss is hard. It's hard for everyone. We hope this realization allows you to shed some of the guilt, frustration, and anger you may feel about yourself and your body.

We hope it allows you to maintain a sense of optimism. We hope that it allows you to maintain that dream, the one of the smaller, healthier, more energetic body. You can build it. We'll show you how.

WHAT BURNED OUT YOUR METABOLISM

We'd like to take you on a journey from birth to the present, showing you the many factors that may have influenced your metabolism. Much of what has disrupted your metabolism and revved up your appetite has probably been beyond your control. Don't get us wrong. Blaming your expanding fat cells on your parents and others won't make those fat cells go away, but blaming that excess fat on yourself won't shrink them down, either. There's nothing to feel guilty about. You haven't been able to change your eating habits or lose weight successfully because, to date, no one has helped you understand the problem.

THE BIRTH OF AN OVERACTIVE APPETITE

Babies cry when they are hungry and stop eating when they are full. Babies do not overeat, and they do not eat because they are sad or lonely. They do not crave foods. They don't feel panicky when in the presence of a Cold Stone Creamery. They eat when they need nourishment, and they stop eating when they've had enough.

Wouldn't it be nice if this natural sense of appetite control lasted? It can. Some babies do grow into children and then adults who eat when they are hungry and stop eating when they've consumed what their bodies need. However, these are rare individuals. The vast majority of us inhabit bodies that make us feel hungry when we should really feel full. The vast majority of us, after finishing a huge holiday meal, will still find room for pie or ice cream, even if our stomachs are pressing against our waistbands.

Why do we reach for the second plateful of pasta even though logic tells us that the first plateful was more than enough? We do so because our natural sensations of hunger and fullness are not working correctly, and the problem may start in infancy. A study completed at the University of Glasgow looked at thousands of children and determined that breastfed babies were 30 percent less likely to grow up into obese children and adults than children who were bottle fed. Why? Breastfeeding encourages babies to nurse only when hungry and to stop nursing when they are full. When babies nurse, they stay in control of the flow of breast milk. Once their stomachs send their brains the "I'm satisfied" signal, they stop nursing. When they are very hungry and want more, they suckle for a longer period of time and more often, which encourages the milk ducts in the breasts to make more milk. When they are less hungry, they suckle less, and breast milk supplies diminish. As a result, they stay in touch with their natural appetite control signals.

Bottle feeding, however, can override these signals. Many parents encourage babies to finish their bottles. A satisfied baby may turn his or her face away from the bottle, but a parent might insert the nipple back into the baby's mouth and even wiggle the bottle back and forth to regain the baby's interest. If the baby takes the bottle again, it's usually not because of hunger, but rather out of curiosity. (So if you do bottle feed, be aware of your baby's body language. When he or she turns away from the nipple, take the bottle away.)

If a baby continually takes the bottle out of curiosity rather than hunger, he or she eventually gets used to the sensation of being too full. Some parents also opt to feed their babies who are crying out of fussiness or discomfort rather than hunger, conditioning the baby to eat emotionally later in life. Problems may have worsened for you when your parents introduced you to your first foods, especially if they fed you sweetened commercial baby foods and encouraged you to keep eating, even if you were turning your head away from the spoon.

THE ORIGIN OF YOUR SWEET TOOTH

As you grew to adulthood, sugar and other sweeteners probably became a dietary staple. Americans today are now consuming 14 percent more sugar, high-fructose corn syrup, and other sweeteners than they did in 1965, with most of us eating more than 20 teaspoons a day. We're eating more sugar than ever before in history, but our bodies have not evolved to handle the increase.

These teaspoons, by the way, rarely come straight from the sugar bowl. They come from processed foods and beverages. Some sources are obvious, such as cakes, cookies, and other sweet desserts. Others are not. You'll find sugar and other sweeteners in flavored yogurt, granola bars, canned or jarred fruit, fruit bars, bran muffins, and breakfast cereal. Even hot dogs, their buns, and ketchup contain added sugar.

Many convenience foods are loaded with added sugars, and many busy people turn to these foods for quick meal options. Consider that some brands of peanut butter, jelly, bread, bologna, breakfast bars, granola bars, canned chili, and canned fruit in syrup all contain added sugar! Sugar or another sweetener is often added to fast foods such as pizza, sandwiches, and even breakfast items. You probably realize that sweetened breakfast cereals contain sugar, but you might be surprised at how much: up to 15 grams of sugar per ounce. And many foods that you might never suspect actually do have added sugar. A fast food biscuit with sausage, according to the USDA, usually has about 1.7 grams of added sugar. A fast food cheese and bacon griddle cake sandwich? It has 9 grams. We think you'll be quite surprised at the vast number of foods that contain added sugar and other sweeteners. Sneak a peek at the "Stealth Sugar" list on page 20. Amazed? We were, too.

And that's just a short list of the foods that most people don't typically think of as being sweet. Desserts and sweet beverages pile on even more of the sweet stuff. You may also have more sugar in the

---

Q: *What are "added sugars"?*

A: Traditionally, sugar has referred to the sweet, white stuff we get from the sugarcane plant. When we see the phrase "added sugars" on a processed food, however, these "sugars" don't always come from that source. Since 1967, they increasingly have come from a sweetener made from corn, called high-fructose corn syrup (HFCS). Added sugars also include brown sugar, dextrose, fruit juice concentrate, honey, maltodextrin, invert sugar, malt syrup, lactose, maltose, molasses, and more. These encourage us to prefer sweet foods—and they have the potential to wreak havoc on blood sugar control.

STEALTH SUGAR

Do you think of the following foods as sweet? We didn't think so, but these foods, among many others, all contain added sugar.

Aunt Jemima original pancake mix

Aunt Jemima whole wheat blend pancake mix

Bush's Best light red kidney beans

Ensure (all products)

Healthy Choice split pea and ham soup

Jif peanut butter

Oscar Mayer hard salami

Oscar Mayer ready to serve bacon

Oscar Mayer shaved turkey breast

Pepperidge Farm soft 100% whole wheat very thin sliced bread

PowerBar performance bars

Progresso dark red kidney beans

form of soft drinks, candy, and cupcakes. If you're active, you've probably been encouraged to load up on sugary sports drinks, energy bars, and other foods before and after you exercise. Television commercials and programming also urge you to eat candy bars and energy bars after exercise, to replace the energy you burn. The ironic part is that most of us do not exercise long enough to burn the calories in the energy bars.

And so grows your tolerance for sweet flavors. These regular sugar fixes may also continue to unravel your natural appetite control systems. Candy, soft drinks, and other foods that contain a lot of sugar are quickly digested and absorbed. This dumps a lot of glucose into your bloodstream at once, causing the pancreas to overproduce insulin, which causes blood sugar to drop quickly. Although eating sugary foods will temporarily turn off appetite fast, hunger returns quickly and very strongly.

This all disrupts your metabolism. You eat sugar and experience a short-lived exhilaration and energy as your adrenal glands produce the stress hormone adrenaline. This hormone drops quickly, so you feel fatigued. You eat more sugar and rise some, only to drop deeper into exhaustion. Each sugar hit gives you a little bounce, followed by a bigger crash.

These bounces and crashes may not have been as pronounced when you were very young and your metabolism was still healthy. Over time, however, as you ate more sugar and as your metabolism became more imbalanced, these sugar highs and lows probably intensified, setting you up not only for weight gain, but also for developing stomach upset, diabetes, heart disease, osteoporosis, and other diseases. It used to take 15 to 20 years for steady consumption of sugar and other sweeteners to trigger conditions such as type 2 diabetes. That's why we used to call type 2 diabetes "adult onset" diabetes: It only affected adults. Now we're seeing type 2 diabetes in children as young as age 6.

Of the various types of corn that are added to processed foods, high-fructose corn syrup (HFCS) is the most prevalent and most problematic. The food industry learned how to turn corn into high-fructose corn syrup in the 1970s. HFCS is made by processing corn-starch into glucose (a form of sugar) and then using enzymes and very high heat to convert the glucose into fructose. The result is a sweet and clear syrup. High-fructose corn syrup is less expensive than sugar, which is why this synthetic sweetener has been replacing sugar as the sweetener of choice in processed foods. Most sports drinks and soft

GOOD FOODS GONE BAD

In the 1920s, Sir Frederick Banting studied the incidence of diabetes in sugar-cane workers, who nibbled on sugarcane as they worked. None of the workers had diabetes. Surprised? Many people are, but there's a good explanation for these counterintuitive study results. Sugarcane is a complete food. It's a plant, after all, and most plant foods are good for us. In addition to sucrose, sugar-cane houses a number of minerals, most notably chromium, that help stabilize blood sugar.

When sugarcane is processed into table sugar, it loses 93 percent of its chromium, 89 percent of its manganese, 98 percent of its cobalt, 83 percent of its copper, 98 percent of its zinc, and 98 percent of its magnesium. Consuming pure refined sugar may also cause your body to excrete chromium, which, ironically, triggers sugar cravings. This mineral loss is typically what happens in the processing of any food, including bread.

FOODS THAT CONTAIN CORN

We're willing to bet you wouldn't expect to find corn (cornstarch, corn syrup, or corn oil) in the following foods, among many others, but it's definitely there:

A1 Steak Sauce

Buitoni Alfredo sauce

Buitoni marinara sauce

Carnation Instant Breakfast, no sugar added, various flavors

Ensure (all products)

Fiber One cereal

Good Seasons salad dressing

Hellmann's Canola Cholesterol Free Mayonnaise

Hellmann's Dijonnaise

Morningstar Farms Garden Veggie Patties

Nestlé Good Start DHA and ARA formulas

Oscar Mayer beef franks, light

Oscar Mayer bologna, light

Perdue breaded chicken nuggets

Post Select Banana Nut Crunch cereal

Reddi-wip

Sabra Luscious Lemon Hummus

Taco Bell flour tortillas

Total Whole Grain Cereal

drinks, for example, no longer contain sugar; they are sweetened with high-fructose corn syrup. You'll find HFCS in sweet foods such as packaged cookies, jams, fruit drinks, and colas. You'll also find it in foods that do not taste sweet: salad dressings, pasta sauces, ketchup, peanut butter, bread, and protein bars. It's even in cough syrup.

Natural fructose is not bad for you when consumed in moderation and along with foods that contain protein and fat. Most people, however, are consuming way too much of this sweetener, mostly in the form of soft drinks and other processed foods. Unlike sugarcane, HFCS does not stimulate leptin release or suppress levels of the hunger hormone ghrelin. When you consume a high number of calories from high-fructose corn syrup, those calories come in, but your satiety hormones fail to flip the switch in your brain that turns off hunger.

Researchers at the University of California have determined that fructose is more likely to be converted into body fat than are other types of sugar. Overweight people who ingested large amounts of this sweetener were more likely to gain still more weight—particularly in the abdomen—than were overweight people who ingested the same amount of regular table sugar.

Large amounts of HFCS also raise your cholesterol levels, increase your insulin levels, and put you at greater risk for high blood pressure, heart disease, and diabetes. Too much HFCS can predispose you to developing gout (high uric acid levels) and kidney disease. Consider the following diseases thought to be triggered or worsened by consuming large amounts of high-fructose corn syrup:

Diabetes. Researchers at Rutgers University in New Brunswick, New Jersey, have shown that soft drinks sweetened with high-fructose corn syrup contain high amounts of reactive carbonyls (a type of free radical) that, when consumed, trigger cell damage that can lead to diabetes. Equally damning, researchers at Harvard have shown that people who consume high amounts of HFCS-sweetened beverages (such as soft drinks) had elevated blood levels of uric acid. Uric acid drives down levels of nitric oxide. Low levels of nitric oxide render the hormone insulin less effective, so the pancreas must make more of it to control blood sugar. In a series of studies done on rats, Harvard researchers showed that high amounts of fructose—and not other types of sugars—induced high insulin, high triglycerides, and high uric acid levels. They also showed that low uric acid levels countered the symptoms of metabolic syndrome.

Finally, researchers at Tufts University have shown that people who drink two or more soft drinks (which are usually sweetened with high-fructose corn syrup) daily were more likely to have higher insulin levels than people who did not consume these drinks.

Heart disease. Body cells readily burn glucose and not fructose. For this reason, fructose first travels to the liver, where it is converted into triglycerides (a type of fat that raises the risk for heart disease and

CORN OIL: THE WHOLE TRUTH

Found in the germ of the corn kernel, corn oil is mostly composed of polyunsaturated fats. This type of fat is called an omega-6 fatty acid, and research shows that eating too much omega-6 can throw off the body's metabolic balance. Diets high in omega-6 fats have been shown to increase inflammation, raising the risk for heart disease and cancer.

FOODS THAT CONTAIN HIGH-FRUCTOSE CORN SYRUP

This sweetener has made its way into most processed foods, including the following (among many others):

Aunt Jemima lite syrup

Breakstone's/Knudsen Cottage Doubles

Campbell's pork & beans

Campbell's tomato soup

Carbonated beverages such as Coca-Cola and 7Up

Claussen Pickles Bread 'n Butter Chips

Colombo Light yogurt, Juicy Peach

Dannon yogurt

Ensure (all products)

Fig Newtons

Freihofer's 100% Whole Wheat bread

Gerber Graduates Zwieback Toast

Kellogg's All-Bran Extra Fiber

Kellogg's Rice Krispies and Corn Flakes, original

Kellogg's Special K cereal

Ken's salad dressings

Kraft barbecue sauces

Kraft salad dressings

Lea & Perrins Worcestershire sauce

Lean Cuisine Chicken à l'orange

Miracle Whip

Motts Classic applesauce

Nabisco 100 calorie packs

Ocean Spray Cranberry Juice Cocktail

Oreos

Pepperidge Farm breads

Shake 'n Bake, Italian

Shake 'n Bake, Ranch and Herb Crusted

Skinny Cow ice cream

Stove Top stuffing

Stroehmann Dutch Country 12 Grain bread

Teddy Grahams

Wheat Thins

Yoplait Light yogurt, Red Raspberry

diabetes), and then circulates in the bloodstream. Rat studies done at the University of California at Davis show that overconsumption of fructose tends to nudge triglycerides upward.

Premature aging. The high-fructose corn syrup in barbecue and other types of sauces causes cooked food to brown seven times faster. This browning reaction creates harmful toxic by-products called advanced glycation end products (AGEs), which increase inflammation and oxidative stress, both of which damage your health.

GI distress. In a study at the University of Kansas in Kansas City, 15 participants drank 25- and 50-gram doses of crystalline fructose (another common food sweetener made from corn). These dosages are common in many processed foods. After the 25-gram dose, more than half of the adults had evidence of fructose malabsorption such as gas, abdominal pain, and loose stools. More than two thirds did after consuming the 50-gram dose.

FLOUR: GOING AGAINST THE GRAIN

Our ancient ancestors probably were much more active than we are today, and they probably did not eat as much flour because of the effort it took to make. Although some cultures certainly relied on specific types of whole grain foods—such as rice and millet in Asian countries, oats in Germany, and barley in the Middle East—it wasn't until the Industrial Revolution that humans began increasingly turning wheat into flour and using it to make bread and pancakes. Advances in milling techniques in the 1800s made refined wheat flour affordable and prevalent. White bread infiltrated the food supply. So did white pasta, refined pancake mixes, and more. These foods were cheap, cooked quickly, and were considered superior to their whole grain counterparts. Because refined grains lack the fiber and nutrient-rich germ and bran, however, they tend to raise blood sugar and insulin levels, trigging hunger, fat storage, and weight gain.

Many grain-based foods are so refined that they've lost all of their initial nutrient value. Worse, refined foods made from flour are easy to overeat. Think about the foods that cause you to lose control. We doubt that meat, fish, or eggs top the list. Do you have a hard time holding yourself to a 2.5-ounce serving of pasta? Can you stop at one crusty bread roll? Can you eat just three crackers or chips?

You probably eat more grain servings than your body needs. In ancient cultures, whole grains were an accent to a meal that consisted of meat or fish and lots of vegetables. In the United States after the 1970s, refined grains became the meal centerpiece, one that was accented with a vegetable garnish and a little meat.

In the 1970s, for example, the U.S. government's Four Food Groups recommended no more than 4 servings of carbohydrate-rich grains a day. Yes, you read that correctly. The government recommended just 4 servings, and all of these servings were supposed to come from whole grains. In the 1990s, the government's Food Guide Pyramid recommended 6 to 11 servings of bread, cereal, and pasta, with no emphasis on whether or not these servings came from whole foods. In 2003, Americans were eating, on average, 10 servings of grains a day. At the same time, we suddenly began consuming more total calories, by more than 400 a day. Grains did not displace other dietary calories; they added to them.

Eating a meal that's high in refined carbohydrates and low in fat and protein affects insulin and blood sugar the same way eating a candy bar does. It causes blood sugar to rise quickly, triggering your pancreas to pump out too much insulin. As insulin levels rise, and as your body ignores its signal, it directs more fat into fat cells and makes you feel hungry again, even if you have just eaten.

MEAT: NOT WHAT IT USED TO BE

Since the 1960s, most meat has come from factory farms. Animals are usually raised in feed lots, where they are crammed into a small space with little ability to move. Instead of grazing on their natural diets of grass and shrubs, most factory-farmed cattle, for instance, eat grain, soy, and corn. This unnatural diet changes the nutritional value of the meat, making it higher in pro-inflammatory fats and lower in heart-healthy fats such as omega-3 fatty acids and conjugated linoleic acid (CLA). Grain-fed beef is also lower in vitamin E, beta-carotene, and vitamin C, important antioxidants that protect your body against serious illnesses such as prostate cancer.

Factory-farmed meat usually also contains trace amounts of antibiotics. With animals crowded together in small lots, diseases spread rapidly. To combat disease, ranchers routinely give antibiotics to livestock, even when the animals display no signs of illness. The antibiotics, by

SOFT DRINKS: THE WHOLE TRUTH

Total soft-drink consumption has increased by 300 percent since the 1950s. Two cans of soda contain 24 teaspoons of sugar in the form of high-fructose corn syrup. This amount of soda has been shown to reduce white blood cell function by 92 percent, an immunity drop that lasts as long as 5 hours.

the way, also make animals gain weight, possibly by killing their intestinal bacteria. The problem is that the antibiotics make their way into an animal's fat and muscle tissue. The farming industry, of course, will tell you that there are no antibiotics left in meat by the time animals go to slaughter. However, the Food and Drug Administration has admitted that meat and poultry are not routinely tested for antibiotic residues and that antibiotics almost undoubtedly end up in the meat you purchase at the store. The agency is generally short staffed and under-funded, which prevents it from being everywhere it should. The scientists at the FDA have also mistakenly assumed that antibiotics in our food supply are harmless.

They're not. If the meat you eat is laced with antibiotics, your intestinal flora may have gotten out of balance. Small but regular doses of antibiotics may have killed off levels of beneficial bacteria in your intestines, allowing yeast and harmful bacteria to proliferate. Researchers at Washington University in St. Louis have shown that people who are overweight tend to have higher amounts of unhealthy bacteria in their intestines than people who are not overweight. The researchers suspect that low amounts of healthful bacteria coupled with high amounts of the wrong types of bacteria create an environment that allows more calories to be absorbed from all of the foods you eat. If you've ever wondered why some people seem to be able to eat more food without gaining weight, this is your answer. They probably have a better balance of bacteria that blocks the absorption of some of the calories that they consume.

Low doses of antibiotics also tend to create antibiotic-resistant superbugs, and various studies have shown that these remain in the meat. When you eat this tainted meat, you also ingest the bugs and introduce them into your GI tract. Although not everyone ends up with an imbalanced GI tract from eating trace amounts of antibiotics every day, most people do.

FOODS THAT CONTAIN SOY

The following foods and brands, among many others, contain soy flour, soy protein isolate, or soybean oil.

Banquet Brown 'N Serve turkey sausage

Benecol spread and other margarines

Buitoni Herbed Chicken Tortellini

Celentano Eggplant Parmigiana

Country Crock Side Dishes, Deluxe Macaroni and Cheese

DiGiorno Pizza

Eggo Nutri-Grain blueberry frozen waffles

Ensure shakes

Fig Newtons

French's Original French Fried Onions

Goldfish crackers, cheddar

Goldfish pretzels

Hellmann's Real Mayonnaise

Hidden Valley salad dressings

I Can't Believe It's Not Butter! spread

Kashi GOLEAN Crunch

Kashi GOLEAN original 7 Grain waffles

Knorr chicken bouillon cubes and dry sauces

Kraft salad dressings

Lean Cuisine Deluxe Pizza

Lean Pockets

LUNA bars

Microwave popcorn

Mrs. Paul's Healthy Selects fish sticks

Nabisco 100 Calorie Snack Packs

Old London croutons

Oreos

Pepperidge Farm Milano cookies

Ry Krisp sesame crackers

Skinny Cow ice cream

Sociables

South Beach Grilled Chicken Caesar Wrap

StarKist, Chicken of the Sea, and Bumble Bee canned tuna

Taco Bell Salsa Con Queso, medium

Teddy Grahams

Thomas' Hearty Grains English muffins

Triscuits, Deli-Style Rye

Wheat Thins

Wheatsworth Stone Ground Wheat Crackers

Wish-Bone salad dressings

GOOD FOODS GONE BAD

Some of the antibiotics fed to farm animals end up in manure that is then used as fertilizer for crops. According to a study completed by the University of Minnesota, crops grown in antibiotic-rich manure absorb these substances into their leaves and fruit. The scientists found antibiotics in corn, potatoes, and lettuce grown in manure-treated soil.

NOT SOY GOOD

In the early 1900s, soy was not a major U.S. crop. It now covers 72 million farmland acres. It's used in animal feed, flavorings, preservatives, sweeteners, emulsifiers, and meat extenders. To mask its beanlike taste, it's often mixed with artificial flavorings, some of which may be unhealthy, too.

Without ever eating a soybean or slice of tofu, you probably consume more soy every day than most Asians consume in a week. By some estimates, soy may be in as much as 60 percent of processed foods, including commercially prepared hamburgers, refried beans, and some brands of canned tuna. It's commonly used as a meat extender and fat reducer in school lunches. Soy oil is used to make many types of margarine. It's also used in commercially prepared cookies, crackers, and baked goods. Soy protein is used to make commercially prepared veggie burgers, pasta sauces, energy bars, and other prepared foods. Soy flour is added to breakfast cereal and pasta. And, because we feed soy to livestock, it has made its way into the meat we eat. It's even in chocolate bars, as well as many processed foods that are marketed as low carb. For an eye-opening list of foods that contain added soy, see "Foods That Contain Soy" on the opposite page.

All of this soy isn't so good. Not many years ago, soy was promoted as a superfood that could reduce the risk of breast cancer, heart disease, and more. It was thought that the substances called isoflavones (specifically genistein and daidzein) in soy promoted health by acting like a weakened form of estrogen in the body. Of course at that time, we also thought that estrogen was a wonder hormone that acted like the fountain of youth. We now know better. As it turns out, some estrogen—when in balance with other hormones—is good, but more isn't better.

In post-menopausal women, estrogen therapy has been linked with an increased risk of heart disease.

Excess soy also impairs fertility and lowers sex drive. In fact, Buddhist monks eat a lot of tofu specifically to reduce their sex drive! Research from Harvard shows that men who consume the most soy tend to have the lowest sperm counts.

In young girls, too much soy can trigger early puberty, causing fertility and hormonal problems later in life. According to the National Institutes of Health (NIH), early puberty can be seen in girls as young as 6. In grown women, too much estrogen causes breast tenderness, decreased sex drive, increased fat storage, fatigue, foggy thinking, and PMS. It may also raise the risk for estrogen-dependent cancers, such as breast, endometrial, and ovarian cancers. In men, it can cause breast tissue growth, prostate enlargement, weight gain, bloating, mood swings, irritability, headaches, fatigue, depression, and hypoglycemia (low blood sugar). It can also lead to prostate, breast, endometrial, and testicular cancers.

Q: *Isn't soy heart healthy?*

A: Studies have refuted this claim, and even early studies that found a connection between soy and heart health did so only in people with very high cholesterol levels (above 250 mg/dl).

Because of its presence in nearly all processed foods, some experts estimate that we may be eating as much as 100 grams of soy protein a day—or 600 milligrams of isoflavones—which is an estrogen dose comparable to a birth control pill.

This is an estrogen overload. Worse, soy also suppresses other hormones, including testosterone and progesterone. And it contains substances called goitrogens that also depress thyroid function. This lowers your metabolism and encourages fat storage.

Fact: Soy isn't the only source of excess estrogens we're exposed to. Synthetic estrogens are injected into cattle and other animals to increase their growth and egg and milk production. The burning of fossil fuels, especially petroleum, produces a type of air pollution that contains xenoestrogens that we breathe continually. These chemicals are also in bug spray, many types of plastic containers, spermicide, detergents, and personal care products.

Q: *How can Asians eat so much soy and remain thin?*

A: Asians don't actually eat as much soy as many people think. For her book *The Whole Soy Story* (New Trends Publishing, 2005), Kaayla T. Daniel, PhD, researched the eating habits of people in China, Thailand, Korea, Vietnam, Indonesia, Mongolia, and Japan. She found that most Asians consume only about 1.5 percent of their calories from soy products such as miso, tempeh, and tofu. They primarily get their protein not from soybeans, but from fish, pork, and chicken.

Keith saw these eating habits firsthand when he lived in Japan while in high school. While there, he noticed that the Japanese ate soy in the form of small chunks of tofu or tempeh, and as miso seasoning. They don't process it and put it into every product they eat.

NO REST FOR THE WEARY

In addition to these various dietary imbalances, you may not get enough sleep. In its "2007 Sleep in America Poll," the National Sleep Foundation determined that most women get less quality sleep than experts recommend. Consider:

- Seven in 10 American women say they frequently experience a sleep problem.
- Six in 10 say they get a good night's sleep only a few nights per week.
- Three in 10 say they have used a sleep aid at least a few nights a week.

This lack of quality sleep is not only a woman's issue—a 2002 poll found that almost 40 percent of *all* Americans get less than 7 hours of sleep each weeknight and an equal percentage are so sleepy during the day that it interferes with daily activities.

Sleep deprivation has a direct impact on our waistlines. One in three women who experience sleep problems almost every night are obese, compared with one in five women who have trouble sleeping just a few nights a month. How many of us have said, "I'll be able to stay awake a little bit longer if I just eat these pretzels (or another snack food)"? Sleep deprivation alters levels of many hormones, including serotonin and leptin. This makes you feel hungrier during the day, strengthening cravings for starchy carbohydrates and sweets. This effect can begin even during childhood: a study completed in Japan determined that 6- and 7-year-olds who slept less were more likely to become obese than their peers who went to bed earlier and slept longer. Children who slept fewer than 8 hours were nearly three times as likely to become obese as children who got 10 or more hours.

It's not necessarily that you're actively trying to stay awake. The problem is more subtle and may involve any or all of the following.

Sleep problems. Sleep apnea and other diagnosable sleep problems affect up to 40 percent of adult women and up to 10 percent of kids. (These sleep problems are becoming more common with the rise in childhood obesity.)

Caffeine consumption. It takes 6 or more hours for half of the caffeine in a food or beverage to leave your body. That means that half of the caffeine consumed at dinner will still be affecting sleep at midnight.

Television watching. The hormone melatonin regulates our circadian clock, with melatonin levels dropping during daylight and rising in the evening to signal sleep. Watching television, working at a computer, or playing video games before bed may disrupt melatonin production by emitting low levels of light and radiation that stop the brain from turning on melatonin production. One Italian study of 75 children in junior high determined that children denied TV, computers, and video games for 1 week experienced a 30 percent rise in melatonin levels.

THE STAGES OF METABOLIC IMBALANCE

When you're young, sugar, high-fructose corn syrup, and other additives may not affect your metabolism that much. Over time, however, poor eating habits pack a stronger metabolic punch as your health progresses through the following three stages.

Metabolic overdrive. When you are stressed, you're in overdrive. When you toss back a triple-shot espresso, you're in overdrive. When you exercise beyond your body's capabilities, you're in overdrive. Overdrive is how you speed up the metabolism. This confuses a lot of people, because if they are struggling with excess weight, they assume that they *want* to speed up their metabolism.

This isn't always the case. Staying in overdrive too often can outstrip your metabolic resources. Stress and lack of sleep, for example, cause the adrenal glands to overproduce the stress hormone cortisol and keep levels elevated. When cortisol increases, so does blood glucose, to provide your muscles with fuel should you need to run fast. The problem is that your muscle cells don't need the glucose when you are responding to emotional stress or lack of sleep, so the hormone insulin increases to shuttle the excess glucose into your fat cells—usually the ones in your abdomen. In an overspent state, insulin does this too efficiently. Too much insulin causes blood glucose to drop too quickly. You crave the one thing that can quickly raise blood glucose: sugar. If you turn to sugar and fat—as most people under stress do—glucose rises, insulin rises, glucose falls. You're hungry again.

Overdrive can also result from eating a lot of sugar, HFCS, and refined foods. In this case, blood sugar rapidly rises and falls, and so does insulin. To compensate for the volatility of rapid rises and falls in sugar and hormones, the metabolism runs fast. In fact, many of my patients who have hypoglycemia (low blood sugar) are fairly slender. It's not until they progress to the "metabolic resistance stage" that they start to gain weight.

As overdrive progresses, the problem magnifies. When insulin levels remain high too long and too often, your brain and muscle cells eventually stop responding. Rather than soaking up blood sugar, muscle cells ignore rises in insulin. Your body starts conserving calories, and you see the results in your gut. Your abdomen grows. Even when you cut calories or portions, you can't seem to get rid of the spare tire or love handles. Meet metabolic resistance, also known as Syndrome X and metabolic syndrome; it puts you at risk for and can also lead to diabetes or polycystic ovarian syndrome, a condition in which women develop high levels of male hormones, cysts in their ovaries, and, frequently, infertility.

Metabolic resistance. High cortisol levels cause fat to be deposited in your abdomen, and insulin and cortisol rise and stay elevated. In the case of insulin, your muscle cells now don't recognize its signal. Once your cells stop responding to insulin (called insulin resistance), your pancreas must produce 10 times as much of the hormone to shuttle sugar into cells. Your brain doesn't recognize increases in insulin either, so it never responds by turning off your appetite. As a result, blood glucose is even more erratic than during metabolic overdrive, alternating from very high highs to very low lows, and you're constantly hungry. High insulin levels tend to lower levels of other important hormones, too, which can erode health in many additional ways.

Your sleep is probably starting to become erratic. You may feel okay when you are at work and under stress, but you crash when you get home or go on vacation. Elevated levels of cortisol during the over-spending stage have now taken a toll on various bodily tissues, slowing metabolism through a loss of muscle mass, impairing digestion, and weakening immunity.

Metabolic burnout. Your adrenals or pancreas or both can't keep overproducing hormones, so they eventually hit a zero balance (or are in the red). Your adrenals may run out of funds first, then your pancreas. When the adrenals don't secrete enough cortisol, you feel tired. When the pancreas doesn't make enough insulin, you have official diabetes, although you've been developing it for years. Other parts of the body start to break down during this stage. Yeast will

Pamela Lamba **Lost 8 Pounds**

I met Dr. Berkowitz through my business as a pharmaceutical sales rep. Every few months I'd bring him samples of insulin. During these visits, I started asking him about the type of medicine he practiced, and he told me something that I found really interesting: He said he was often able to help his diabetic patients get their blood sugar down without treating them with insulin. I didn't, at the time, think it applied to me personally—save for the fact that I sold a product that he didn't have much use for!

Then I started to feel out of sorts. I was only 32, but I could not get out of bed in the morning. I was tired and depressed, and I didn't know why. At 5 foot 8 inches tall and 142 pounds, I was not overweight. I'd been thin my entire life. I just didn't feel right.

Fast-forward 2 years. Every little task felt difficult. My relationship with my significant other was falling apart. I did not have the energy to exercise. My friends kept telling me, "You are so young. You should be more healthy." My hair was falling out in clumps. It was horrifying. I was desperate.

I went to a series of doctors who prescribed one medication after another to treat my thyroid, balance my hormones, control my blood sugar, and treat my depression and insomnia—and they kept increasing the drug doses. I couldn't imagine taking this extensive cocktail of medicines for the rest of my life. They were treating my symptoms. They were not curing me.

more easily colonize the digestive tract and the thyroid begins to break down.

LET'S BALANCE YOUR METABOLIC MECHANISMS

Now you understand why and how your body is working against your efforts. This is why willing yourself to lose weight just doesn't work. You can't just eat less and exercise more. You need a different approach, one that helps undo the damage inflicted in the past. That's exactly what our approach is all about.

In Chapter 3, you'll learn how and why eating a balanced low-carbohydrate diet that allows you to occasionally splurge will actually help turn down hunger and cravings, turn up fat burning, and improve energy and mood.

One morning, I remembered Dr. Berkowitz and what he'd said about his patients with diabetes. If he could help them control their blood sugar without insulin, maybe he could help me. I made an appointment. He ran a series of tests that revealed that my blood sugar was spiking from very low to very high. He gave me an eating plan and some supplements. He didn't judge me in any way. I felt as if he were my partner in improving my health.

At first, I struggled with the dietary plan because I'm Indian and my traditional diet includes lots of rice, lentils, and bread. I included some of the more traditional fare, such as chickpeas. It took sheer willpower to get through the first few days. Once, in the beginning, I slipped up and allowed myself to eat a chocolate bar. Then I ate three more. The next morning I felt so tired and so gross. It helped me make the connection between my diet and my health, and I never slipped up again after that.

My boyfriend was so supportive; he did the diet with me. Within a week I felt 50 percent better, and within a month I was 8 pounds lighter. I found I preferred this way of eating. I felt as if a horrible fog had lifted.

Now I'm off almost all of my meds. I wake up every morning ready to face the day. Before this plan, I used to rush home from work so I could lie on the couch. Now, three or four times a week, I go to the gym after work. My relationship with my boyfriend has improved, and I am more fun and have more energy. I feel amazing. I have my life back.

HOW HEALTHY IS YOUR METABOLISM?

If you answer yes to any of the following questions, your metabolism is out of balance.

Do you feel tired all the time?

Do you wake frequently at night?

Do you feel hungry between meals, even if you've just eaten?

Do you crave candy, soda, or coffee, especially in the mid-afternoon?

If you answered yes to at least one of these questions, you have some of the classic symptoms of a metabolic disadvantage. This underlying medical condition is blocking your every attempt to lose weight. Now that you know what's wrong, you're ready to fix the problem.

HOW YOU'LL LOSE
THE WEIGHT

If you follow the diet, lifestyle, and supplement recommendations we suggest, you'll lose up to 10 pounds a month until you reach your goal. You'll bring your metabolism back into balance, reducing the extreme hunger and fatigue that have plagued you in the past. You'll also improve your health in a multitude of ways. You'll reduce artery-clogging cholesterol and blood pressure. Your risk for cancer and diabetes will drop. You may see a reduction in symptoms of other chronic health conditions, such as fibromyalgia, allergies, asthma, and more. You'll feel so good after losing the weight and switching to a healthier lifestyle that you'll never want to go back. You'll stay with it, not because you like how you look or because you're enamored with your new clothing size. Sure, those are great motivators, but you'll stay with it because you'll have so much energy, be in such a good mood, and feel so amazingly fantastic.

Here's how you'll do it.

HOW YOU'LL EAT

Our eating approach will fill you up on fewer calories at the same time that it drives down levels of insulin and other hunger-producing hormones. You'll fill every plate with natural foods that are rich in appetite-suppressing fiber, protein, and fat. By avoiding foods with weight-gain-promoting additives such as soy and various sweeteners, you'll balance key hormones. And you'll learn to head off any carb binges by strategically inserting a "cheat" into your day, at a time when you need it most.

You'll eat according to the following four key nutritional principles:

Principle #1: Make Every Carb Count

We believe in balance, and balanced eating is what it'll take to reach your goal weight. You're reading this book, however, because your body is not in balance, and your eating habits probably aren't either. Until you heal your metabolic disadvantage and lose weight, you'll need to put an end to the hormonal havoc that excess carbohydrates and unhealthy fats have caused. You will temporarily scale back on less nutritious sources of carbohydrates and increase the healthier ones. By modifying your carbohydrate consumption, you will keep extreme blood sugar spikes to a minimum. This allows your pancreas a much needed rest. With blood sugar relatively steady, the pancreas does not need to continually secrete insulin to shuttle that sugar into cells. As insulin levels drop and stay low, it takes stress off organs throughout your body—including your kidneys, heart, liver, thyroid, and adrenals—so these organs can heal.

In one study of low-carb diets, participants were told to restrict carbohydrates, but otherwise eat until they were satisfied. They did not have to count calories or control portions. Another group reduced fat and portions sizes, trying to subtract 500 to 800 calories a day. After 12 weeks, the low-carbohydrate group lost twice as much weight as the low-fat group, and more than double the amount of body fat.

Critics of low-carbohydrate diets will tell you that you can lose weight by cutting back on any of the major macronutrients—protein, fat, or carbs. What do we think? We think it's possible that some people can lose weight simply by cutting back on fat. We also know it's not possible for others. We know this because we've seen these others in our practice. Steven, an executive who works in New York City, is a great example. For most of his life, he dieted off and on, usually going on a very low-fat diet to lose weight. This strategy worked until he was in his late 50s, roughly 50 pounds overweight, and insulin resistant. Steven once again resorted to the weight loss strategy he'd used most of

WHAT ARE CARBS THAT COUNT?

You'll never have to count carb grams on this plan—or fat or protein grams, or calories, or anything, really. We've done the math for you. In the beginning, you'll be on a strict but reasonable carbohydrate budget. As your metabolism comes into balance, you'll get more carbohydrate funds to spend. Eventually, as you approach maintenance, you'll consume a balanced amount of carbohydrates. All of your carbs will be:

- Low in starch and high in fiber. Countless studies have proven that fiber helps blunt the blood sugar swings caused by carb foods. Fiber also protects against colon cancer, reduces cholesterol and risk of heart disease, and feeds the "good" bacteria in your intestinal tract that protect you from dangerous germs and viruses. In every meal, you'll load up on vegetables such as broccoli, spinach, salad greens, Brussels sprouts, cabbage, eggplant, and peppers, among others. These foods are naturally lower in starch and higher in fiber.

- Almost void of additives and preservatives, such as isolated soy protein, high-fructose corn syrup, crystalline fructose, and artificial colors and flavorings.

- As minimally processed as possible. Whole organic fresh fruits are better than skinned, jarred fruit. Raw nuts are better than roasted. Whole grains (barley, quinoa, wild rice, and oats) are better than products made from flour (such as breakfast cereals), even if some of the flour is whole grain flour. This is because most processed foods made from flour (bread, cereals, crackers, and so on) contain a mixture of refined and whole grain flour. If you check the ingredients labels, you'll see that nearly all of these supposedly whole grain foods are much lower in fiber than you may realize.

his life. He lost about 20 pounds, but it wasn't easy. He had to eat almost no fat, and the pounds dropped excruciatingly slowly. Then, his weight loss stalled altogether. It seemed he was eating almost nothing and was hungry all the time, but the weight wouldn't budge.

That's when Steven came to see Valerie. She explained that the high amounts of carbohydrates he was consuming were elevating his insulin levels, working against his efforts to reverse his insulin resistance. She encouraged him to eat more fat and fewer carbs. "I was surprised at some of the things I could eat on this diet. I could have cream cheese and avocado. I could have many foods I loved, but had been trying not to eat over the years. I started eating cheese omelets again, and the weight started rolling off. I was surprised and delighted," he says. His story is a common one at our center. That's why we believe so strongly in what we are telling you to do. We believe in it because it works.

How does it work? Reducing the amount of carbohydrates in your diet enables weight loss in a number of ways. First, you may consume fewer calories because you are no longer insanely hungry! Research shows that:

A low-carbohydrate eating plan turns off your hunger switch. Of the three macronutrients, fat and protein are most satisfying. Both take longer to digest than carbohydrates. As they sit in the stomach and the intestines, they weigh down these organs, stimulating stretch receptors to tell your brain, "Still full down here. No additional food is needed." Fat also does not increase blood sugar as much as protein and carbohydrates can (despite popular belief, some of the protein you consume is converted into blood sugar). This keeps insulin levels low, so fat cells will be more likely to notice small insulin increases and respond by releasing leptin, a hormone that travels to the brain with one loud message: "I'm full."

Carbohydrates, on the other hand, always increase blood sugar, with some types of carbohydrate foods increasing it more than others. This is why you can feel very hungry shortly after eating a large bagel, even though you've consumed as many as 400 calories.

Research published in the *Journal of Nutrition* shows that in addition to normalizing insulin levels, a low-carbohydrate diet reduces hunger in the following ways:

- It makes the brain more sensitive to the fullness hormone leptin.
- It prevents a rise in the hunger hormone ghrelin that is typical with most diets.
- It elevates levels of a hormone called cholecystokinin (CCK) after meals, ensuring that the brain listens to the fullness signals it gives off. When the brain is more sensitive to leptin and insulin signals, it is also more receptive to CCK signals.

End result: Compared to low-fat diets, low-carbohydrate diets flip off your hunger switch earlier during a meal and keep it flipped off for longer after eating. Low-carb plans are particularly effective for people who have metabolic syndrome (high insulin levels coupled with other risk factors such as low HDL). Indeed, in the *Journal of Nutrition* study we mentioned earlier, half of the participants with metabolic syndrome who followed a low-carb diet were cured of the disease.

A low-carb diet promotes fat burning. Cells throughout your body are capable of burning a number of different fuels for energy, including carbohydrates (in the form of blood glucose or muscle glycogen), protein, fat, and ketones (by-products of fat burning). By putting yourself on a carbohydrate budget, you'll consume fewer carbohydrates than your body uses for energy. After 2 or 3 days on our eating plan, your body will have burned through its stores of carbohydrates in your muscles and liver. Once your carbohydrate gas tank reads "empty," insulin drops and stays low. Think of insulin as a switch. When it's high, you burn carbohydrates for energy and store excess calories as fat more easily. When it's low, your body can burn fat rather than storing it, and it will also burn triglycerides—fat in the bloodstream—lowering your risk for heart disease.

A low-carb diet might improve your metabolism. It takes more work for your body to break down protein than to break down carbohydrates. This digestive calorie burning is known as the thermogenic effect of food. The fat-burning boost you get from lowering high insulin levels will also bolster metabolism. Research done at Harvard

CALM YOUR QUALMS ABOUT KETONES

The increase in ketones that results from fat burning can cause minor, short-lived side effects, including dizziness, headache, low energy levels, and weakness. These symptoms simply indicate that your body has become more efficient at burning fat—they are the same sensations that long-distance runners or athletes experience after long periods of exercise. The fact is, every cell in your body is capable of using ketones for energy, and your heart and brain run 25 percent more efficiently on ketones than they do on glucose. Although a low-carbohydrate diet raises ketone levels, the increase is a slight one. Most people—regardless of how they eat—have elevated levels of ketones when they wake in the morning, as a result of their overnight fast. The level of ketones your body produces on a low-carbohydrate diet is only slightly higher than this waking level. It does not even come close to approaching the level that signals danger.

found that people who followed a low-carbohydrate diet were able to eat about 500 more calories a day than participants on a high-carb, low-fat diet and lose just as much weight.

Fiber Makes Our Plan Stick

Fiber is one of the elements that sets our plan apart from other low-carbohydrate approaches you may have tried. In our opinion, it's what makes low carb work.

Fiber is the indigestible part of plant foods. It is not absorbed into the bloodstream. Rather, it travels through your intestine and back to the outside world in your stool. It's housed in the skins, seeds, and pulp of fruit and vegetables and in the bran and germ of grains and legumes. It's what makes food chewy and crunchy, and, in most cases, good for you.

By consuming more fiber-rich carbs, you will support weight loss in the following ways:

You'll feel full sooner after eating. High-fiber foods are chewy, and, as a result, take a long time to eat. This slowed eating pace allows fullness signals from your stomach and intestines the time they need to reach your brain and flip off your hunger switch. Fiber also makes food heavy, weighing down and filling up your stomach. This triggers stretch receptors and nerves to turn off your hunger switch.

Q: *Why is low carb better than low fat for weight loss?*

A: Do you know people who have lost weight and kept it off by following a low-fat, high-carbohydrate diet? We do, too. These diets can work for some people, as long as they follow them in a healthful way (eating real food that is high in fiber and minimally processed). Although low-fat diets can work and be safe, they don't work for everyone. A recent study completed at the University of Connecticut determined that for people with insulin resistance, low-carbohydrate diets are more effective than low-fat diets. In people with healthy metabolisms, either type of diet works effectively, as long as you can stick with it. If your insulin function is in overdrive, however, research shows that a low-carb approach *triples* your weight loss. (Take our quiz in Chapter 5 to find out your metabolic status.)

FIBER: THE WHOLE TRUTH

In 1900, the average American consumed more than 30 percent of daily calories from fiber-rich whole grain foods. Today, that number has dropped to less than 1 percent. Yet, Americans are eating more grains. How can we be consuming less fiber if we're eating more grain? Nearly all of the grain we consume comes from refined wheat flour, which contains little to no fiber.

You'll stay full longer after eating. In your intestines, some types of high-fiber foods turn into a thick glue that slows and in some cases prevents the absorption of calories and sugar. When less sugar enters the bloodstream at once, the pancreas makes less insulin. Lower insulin levels equal lower hunger levels and less fat storage.

You may think, "I won't be eating a lot of carbohydrates, so my blood sugar levels won't matter anyway." That's not true. Your body is capable of converting protein into blood sugar and will do so if you consume a diet rich in protein and low in fiber, carbohydrates, and fat. This drives up insulin levels, even in the absence of carbohydrates, and is *precisely* why many people hit a plateau on typical low-fiber, low-carbohydrate diets. For example, most endocrinologists know that they can't give their diabetic patients a shake composed of 100 percent protein. You only need 1 to 1.5 grams of protein per kilogram of body weight a day to preserve muscle, so the rest gets converted into glucose. When someone with diabetes converts protein into glucose, insulin rises. When people with diabetes consume 100 percent protein on an empty stomach, they get the shakes or feel lightheaded. The body converts the protein into glucose, so glucose rises dramatically, even though they did not consume sugar.

You'll nourish the good bacteria. As we've mentioned, intestinal yeast overgrowth and bacterial imbalances can slow metabolism and trigger health problems. Maintaining a thriving population of probiotics, or beneficial bacteria, in your gut is a very important way to tamp down dangerous bacteria. When you eat fiber, you support your probiotic population because fiber is a "prebiotic," a precursor to food that keeps healthy bacteria alive. Because the typical American diet is so low in fiber, it literally starves these good bacteria, allowing harmful organisms such as yeast (which survive on sugar, not fiber) to flourish.

You'll stay regular. Fiber adds bulk to your stool, which makes it pass through your digestive tract more easily. Although this may not have a direct effect on your weight, you'll feel a heck of a lot better. Your stomach size will also naturally decrease by as much as an inch as excess gas and bloating resolve.

You may have read that you should consume 25 to 30 grams of fiber a day. However, 30 grams of fiber means that only 10 percent of the 300 grams of carbohydrates you eat on a high-carb diet comes from fiber. A better general rule is that your fiber grams should total between 20 and 50 percent of your total carbohydrate grams. On Level 1 of this plan, you'll get between 15 and 20 grams of fiber a day, slightly less than current recommendations but it totals roughly 30 to 40 percent of your carbohydrate intake on this plan. On Level 2, you'll consume 20 to 30 grams of fiber, which comes to 20 to 30 percent of your total carbohydrate consumption. Remember, one of the most important functions of fiber is blood sugar control: Fiber slows the absorption of sugar into the bloodstream. Valerie created the Fiber Scores table on page 99 to help you make food choices that give you the most bang out of your "carbohydrate" buck.

Principle #2: Eat Clean

When we say clean, we're not talking about a lack of dirt. We're talking about food that's free of synthetic additives. We're talking about eating vegetables, meats, eggs, and fruit that are produced naturally. Clean foods do not contain:

- Antibiotic residues
- Hormones (growth hormone)
- Synthetic fats (trans fats, partially hydrogenated oils)
- Additives and preservatives (soy, corn, sweeteners, artificial colors and flavorings)
- Pesticides, herbicides, and pollutants (PCBs, mercury, etc.)

Many additives, preservatives, and other contaminants not only block weight loss but also erode your health. In Chapter 2, you learned how soy, high-fructose corn syrup, sugar, and other additives have played havoc with your metabolism. Because most processed foods contain these additives, you will eat few processed foods on this plan. How can you tell whether a food has been processed? It can be difficult. Here are a few clues.

- Read the label for items listed on this page
- It comes with packaging, such as a box, a can, a bag, or shrink-wrap
- It is made from refined flour (such as cereal, crackers, bread, etc.)

Consider any food that is made from flour (bread, crackers, muffins, pancakes, etc.) or that is not a fresh fruit, vegetable, or animal product a "yellow" food. By that, we're referring to a yellow traffic signal. Slow down, and use caution. Most important, read labels! That's one good thing about nearly all processed foods: They come with a nutrition facts label and ingredients list. If you see any of the following words on the ingredients list, your food contains additives that could interfere with weight loss:

- Crystalline fructose
- Corn oil
- Corn syrup
- Cornstarch
- Dextrose
- High-fructose corn syrup
- Hydrogenated and partially hydrogenated vegetable (usually soybean) oil
- Hydrogenated starch hydrolysate
- Maltodextrin
- Soy grits
- Soy protein concentrate
- Soy protein isolate
- Soy lecithin
- Textured soy protein

We realize that commercially prepared convenience foods are part of our culture and it is almost impossible to completely eliminate them. So to make things as easy as possible, we've done a lot of sleuthing for you. In "Recommended Brands" on page 94, you'll find an extensive list of approved products that are free of unwanted additives or have very minimal amounts. We may not have found every single brand of clean food, but we've certainly found a lot of them. You may find additional brands in your grocery store, too.

Although we can't cite any studies proving that environmental contaminants (such as the mercury, dioxins, and PCBs so common in fish) and food additives (such as the nitrates in lunch meat) result in weight gain, we want you to live a long, healthy life. Anything that interferes with your health will probably interfere with your metabolism. We'd be remiss if we didn't at least caution you against eating the following additives and contaminants:

Nitrates. We caution against eating processed meats (bacon, lunch meat, hot dogs) that contain nitrates, chemicals that have been linked to cancer. Look for nitrate-free brands of lunch meat, smoked foods, and franks.

Mercury and other environmental pollutants. Our rivers and oceans absorb the mercury produced when we drive cars, burn coal to fuel power plants, and incinerate household wastes. They've also become toxic waste dumps for many other industrial pollutants, such as PCBs and dioxin. These harmful chemicals are absorbed into algae and plants that are then eaten by fish. The pollutants become more and more concentrated as they travel up the food chain. Once one of the world's healthiest foods, all wild fish and even some farm-raised varieties are contaminated with disease-promoting chemicals. To reduce your risk of consuming more of these toxins than your body can clear, consume only fish that have been shown to have the lowest levels of mercury (see "The Cleanest Fish on the Planet" on page 52).

Sugar substitutes. According to a report from the Center for Science in the Public Interest, some alternative sweeteners have been associated with health problems. Saccharin and aspartame are suspected carcinogens; stevia is thought to reduce fertility in men and may contribute to birth defects; and sorbitol, malitol, mannitol, and polydextrose cause gas and diarrhea in most people and may adversely affect insulin levels. To reduce your risk of suffering these effects, we recommend you limit the use of and rotate artificial sweeteners, alternating among a few different types rather than staying loyal to just one.

If you think artificial sweeteners have zero calories, think again. Right there on the ingredients label you can see that they contain dextrose or maltodextrin, a cornstarch-based sweetener that adds calories. And, oh yes, a long-term study of thousands of residents in Framingham, Massachusetts, recently determined that people who drank more than one soft drink—diet or regular—a day had an increased risk of developing metabolic syndrome, a cluster of disorders that includes abdominal fat, insulin resistance, and high blood pressure and cholesterol.

It may be that excessively sweet foods—whether they are sweetened with real sugar or with an artificial sweetener—increase cravings for sweets in general. Although you consume few calories from the sweetener, the increased cravings for sweetness may cause you to overeat foods containing sugar or high-fructose corn syrup. So if you sweeten your food with "sugar substitute" packets, keep in mind that these packets do contain about 1 gram of sugar each. In reality, they are not "noncalorie" sweeteners. We understand that you may not be able to completely forgo these sweeteners, but limit them as much as you can.

Pesticide residues. Conventional farmers use more than 400 chemicals to kill weeds, insects, and pests that attack crops. Fruits and vegetables are washed many times before they reach the supermarket, but tests show that pesticide residues linger. Researchers have determined that up to 17 percent of the original pesticide residue remains on produce. These residues are probably harmful to your health, and may interfere with your metabolism.

Does 100 percent of your produce have to be organic? No—especially if you can't afford to pay the higher prices that are often charged for these foods. Use this buying guide:

Best to buy organic: According to the Environmental Working Group, the following foods tend to contain high amounts of pesticide residues: apples, bell peppers, celery, cherries, grapes, nectarines, peaches, pears, potatoes, red raspberries, spinach, and strawberries.

Not as necessary to buy organic: The following foods tend to have little if any pesticide residues: asparagus, avocados, bananas, broccoli, cauliflower, corn, kiwi, mangos, onions, papaya, pineapple, and peas.

Antibiotic, soy, and hormone residues. Organically raised animals are less likely to ingest foods laced with pesticides and are therefore less likely to have pesticide residues in their meat. They are generally free from antibiotic residues and have not been subjected to hormone injections. Animals allowed to graze on grass, bushes, and other natural dietary staples produce meat that is higher in healthful omega-3 fats. Eggs from free-range chickens that eat bugs and other natural foods tend to be higher in the heart- and metabolism-healthy omega-3 fatty acids than eggs from factory-raised hens fed a diet rich in soy.

Principle #3: Eat Real Fat to Burn Fat

Synthetic trans fat (hydrogenated or partially hydrogenated vegetable oil) has been linked to a range of health conditions, including obesity. Although food manufacturers have been reducing their use of trans fats in recent years, the additive still remains in many processed foods.

Real fats are not synthetic. They are found in nature's foods and come from:

- Animals raised on food they were designed to eat (not grain or soy)
- Vegetables
- Fatty fruits such as avocados and olives
- Nuts and seeds
- Olive and coconut oils
- Fish

Here's another way in which we diverge from other low-carb diets you may have tried. Many popular diets tell you to replace carbs with lean protein such as egg whites and skinless chicken breast. They also tell you to refrain from adding fat to your food. In other words, skip the butter and the olive oil. Does this sound like a fun way to eat to you? If it doesn't, that's probably why you couldn't stick with such diets.

You can lose weight—possibly even faster and definitely in a more healthful way—by not concerning yourself with the leanness of the meat you eat or avoiding fatty vegetables such as olives. Eat the meat you want. Go ahead and have real eggs. Put avocado in your salads. Eat the dark meat on that chicken. (You can even have the skin.) Go ahead and have red meat, too. Use real oil on your green salad and real mayonnaise in your tuna salad. Enjoy fat and enjoy it without guilt!

Are you surprised? This advice of ours may make you feel uneasy because you've been conditioned to fear fat. This conditioning stems from the 1980s, when a University of Massachusetts biochemist named J. P. Flatt published research that showed it is rare for the human body

AVOCADOS, THE DAILY INDULGENCE

Many people think of avocados as a fatty food, and they are. But the type of fat in avocados is good for your health, and these fruits also contain an amazing amount of fiber. Consider:

- Their healthful monounsaturated fats have been shown to raise levels of the good HDL cholesterol and drop levels of the bad LDL cholesterol.

- They are a rich source of lutein, an antioxidant thought to promote eye health.

- Avocados contain beta-sitosterol, a plant substance thought to drive down cholesterol levels.

- They are a rich source of 20 vitamins and minerals, including vitamin E, beta carotene, vitamin C, folate, potassium, and iron, which strengthen your immunity and give you more energy.

- Because they are rich in both fiber and fat, they are particularly effective at keeping you going to the bathroom regularly.

- In a study completed at Ohio State University, antioxidant nutrients from avocados stopped the growth of cancerous tumors that led to oral cancer.

If you love avocados, as most of our patients do, go ahead and eat half an avocado (either plain or as guacamole) every day. The creamy texture will satisfy you emotionally and physically.

to convert carbohydrates into body fat. This news, coupled with the fact that fat has nine calories per gram compared with four for carbohydrates and protein, led many dieters to one conclusion: fat makes you fat.

The problem is, the conclusion was false. Harvard's 8-year Nurse's Health Study of more than 41,000 women determined that dietary fat has very little influence on body weight as long as your carbohydrate intake is in balance. Studies that have linked fat consumption with adverse health outcomes did not rule out confounders, such as the nitrates found in some types of meat or synthetic trans fats. What makes humans unhealthy and fat isn't necessarily eating too much fat. It's eating too much period, especially too much trans fats. Every 1 percentage increase in trans fats consumption is accompanied by a weight increase of 2 pounds. A Wake Forest University study determined that monkeys who ate more trans fats gained 30 percent more abdominal fat than monkeys who ate the same percentage of monounsaturated fats (the type of fat found in avocados and olive oil).

As you'll learn in Chapter 4, fat is quite healthy for you, as long as you eat the right types of fat in the right balance. Some fatty acids are essential to life; your body cannot make them. They improve digestion and help us digest vitamins A, D, E, and K, and many fat-soluble minerals and antioxidants.

It's important to eat a variety of different types of fat, including saturated fat. The truth is that trying to eliminate saturated fat from meat and eggs will probably bring you out of balance by causing you to overconsume fats from vegetable oils. Vegetable oils are rich in a type of fat called omega-6 fatty acids. Omega-6 isn't bad for your health or waistline unless you consume too much of it and too little of another type of fat called omega-3 fatty acids. When you eat too many omega-6 fats and too few omega-3 fats, you increase inflammation throughout your body and reduce your body's ability to burn body fat. You'll learn more about this in Chapter 4, because consuming balanced amounts of omega-3 and omega-6 is important for good health. For now, however, it's important to know which foods contain omega-3 fats. Fatty fish, such as salmon, are a great source, but so are eggs and meat, particularly if they are from animals raised on a natural diet rather than a soy- or grain-based diet. Organically raised hens, as we've mentioned, lay eggs that are richer in this healthful fat than conventionally raised hens. Grass-fed beef tends to also be higher in omega-3s than grain-fed beef.

DOES THIS MAKE SENSE?

We've seen news stories that claim chocolate pudding pops have "less fat than you think" and avocados have "more fat than you need." Avocados are a fruit that grows in nature and that have been eaten by humans for thousands of years. They contain a number of health-promoting antioxidants, plus heart-healthy monounsaturated fat, fiber, vitamin K, potassium, folate, vitamin C, and copper. Pudding pops are a relatively recent invention made from refined sugar, high-fructose corn syrup, or both. They contain calories and little to no nutrition. Why on Earth would it be better for you to eat a pudding pop than an avocado, an egg, or a handful of olives?

EGGS COME BACK TO THE TABLE

People shy away from eggs because of outdated research about the dangers of dietary cholesterol and fat. Eggs, as it turns out, are one of the healthiest foods on the planet. The yolks contain lutein and zeaxanthin (antioxidants that protect your eyes from cataracts and blindness) and choline (important in preserving memory). The yolk's B vitamins probably reduce the risk of heart disease by neutralizing a toxic blood chemical called homocysteine. Along with half the egg's protein, the yolk also contains vitamins A, D, and E, along with the minerals iron and zinc. It's true that the yolk contains 212 milligrams of cholesterol. But it's also true that most of the cholesterol from food passes through the gut, without ever making its way into the bloodstream. The yolk may contain all of the fat, but Harvard research has shown that consuming eggs does *not* raise heart disease risk.

Think about it this way: eggs were a dietary staple for our ancient ancestors, whose metabolisms evolved on a diet that included whole eggs, not egg whites. Eggs are a whole food that have been on the planet since the beginning of human life. Does it make sense that we're only supposed to eat part of what's inside? It sure doesn't to us.

Here's where things can get complicated, though. As we've mentioned, because our oceans are polluted you should probably limit your consumption of fish, one of the best sources of omega-3s. We recommend you choose the least-contaminated varieties of fish (see "The Cleanest Fish on the Planet" on page 52). To ensure you get enough omega-3s, we recommend you take a fish oil supplement. You'll learn more about this in Chapter 9.

Principle #4: Add in Indulgences

Okay, so you know this diet plan will help you drop pounds fast and stay healthy. But the problem is, it will only work if you can stick with it. What if you really love ice cream or chocolate or bread? Are you destined to a lifetime of shopping in the plus-size area of the clothing store? In a word, no.

We've seen many of our patients have trouble with the more restrictive low-carb plans—just one taste of a carb could send them over the

THE CLEANEST FISH ON THE PLANET

All fish contain some pollutants, including mercury, which is why we recommend you eat no more than 12 ounces of fish a week. According to U.S. Environmental Protection Agency tests, the following fish have the lowest levels of mercury:

- Shrimp

- Pollock

- Catfish

- Canned Tongol tuna

- Wild salmon (Farmed salmon are also relatively low in mercury, but they are dosed with antibiotics and consume feed containing a pigment that is a suspected carcinogen. This feed is also rich in the remains of fatty fish such as sardines and, as a result, tends to contain contaminants like PCBs and dioxin.)

edge into a binge. By adding the right carbs and essential fiber, the basic nutritional tenets of our program go a long way toward satisfying the carb cravings that can be the undoing of most low-carb dieters. But we know there are some times when the flavor of chocolate or a small bowl of ice cream can make the world seem more manageable. We get that. We wish it weren't so, but we understand. Decades of mental and emotional programming cannot be easily undone with good intentions. And we also know that labeling something "forbidden fruit" only makes it more desirable. Our ultimate goal is to get you to follow the plan for life, and that's never going to work if you can't sustain it for a month or two—or even a week or two—at a time.

That's why you'll be allowed your choice of indulgence foods from day one. Initially, you'll choose a treat, whether it be delicious berries (our favorite!) or bread or chocolate, every day. Then add the foods you most love. Pick one of the following treats:

- ice cream
- starch
- beer and wine
- salty snack
- chocolate

This will allow you to have it all. You can have the weight loss, as well as the considerable health benefits, but you can do away with low-carb deprivation.

The key to this plan is learning *when* to eat your treat. Our patients typically find that late afternoon or late night cravings for sweets have been their undoing. Why is that? Bottom line, they haven't eaten enough—they misjudged how much to eat during dinner or missed an afternoon snack. Their blood sugar dropped and their bodies wanted quick carbs to boost it back up again. With our plan, you'll learn to savor your indulgence foods with or just after meals, rather than separately, to reduce the risk of overeating. You'll piggyback on your meals' blood-sugar-stabilizing fat, fiber, and protein, to ensure that your body will not respond to the extra carbs with dramatic spikes in blood sugar and insulin. No longer will you mindlessly medicate your stress with carbs and just make matters worse—sugar "crash," anyone? With this plan, you'll understand how you can enjoy the treat while you also feel calmer and more satisfied on every level. And that satisfaction will help you stick with this eating plan long enough not only to lose the weight but to reap countless other long-term health benefits as well.

HOW TO LIVE

This isn't just a diet. To lose weight and keep it off, we recommend a total lifestyle change. You must make yourself a top priority. Most important, we recommend you rest your body by reducing stress, getting more sleep, and possibly scaling back or avoiding exercise until you've lost weight and improved your metabolism. This rest is mandatory for optimal adrenal, pancreatic, and thyroid function.

We talked about the importance of sleep in Chapter 2. If you suffer from insomnia or have other sleep issues, you'll find advice for fixing these problems in Chapter 10.

Let's talk about stress. Turning to food when you are under stress and eating when you are not physically hungry are two of the fastest ways to gain weight. Stress also raises levels of the hormone cortisol. High levels of cortisol increase body fat storage, make you feel hungry, and increase cravings for sweets. Cortisol also tends to preferentially direct fat to the abdomen.

Elissa Epel, PhD, a researcher from the University of California at San Francisco, put 59 women in a stressful situation (they were told to complete a task but were not given enough time to get it done) and then asked them to sit in a room that contained different types of snack foods. The women who felt the most stressed from the exercise tended to snack more, and they tended to choose the foods richest in sugar.

You'll find simple and effective stress reduction techniques in Chapter 10.

HOW TO SUPPLEMENT

If we lived in a perfect world and ate perfectly every day, none of us would need supplements. We don't live in a perfect world, however. In the world we live in, our produce is not as nutritious as in years past. It grows in mineral-depleted soil and loses countless nutrients and antioxidants as it is trucked across the country. In the world we live in, most of our animal meat and products come from livestock fed an unnatural diet of grain and soy. This, as we've mentioned, yields meat that is not as nutritious as that from animals fed a natural diet.

It'd be great if you could purchase only organic vegetables at a local farmer's market and find locally raised meat and eggs from small farmers who allowed the animals to graze naturally. It's a great goal, but few of us manage to do it all the time. All of this makes supplements a must. They help fill the nutritional gaps created by less than perfect food sources and eating habits. Supplements also help fix underlying metabolic issues—such as insulin resistance, yeast overgrowth, adrenal fatigue, and more—that tend to slow or block weight loss.

In Chapter 9, you'll find a list of the supplements we recommend.

WHAT TO EXPECT

By eating differently, building in indulgences, changing your lifestyle, and taking the right supplements, you'll remove your barriers to weight loss. You'll lose an accelerated amount of weight in the first week or two on this plan. You may lose up to 10 pounds in just 1 week. Expect this rapid weight loss to taper off; some of it is water and stored carbohydrates. Once your body adjusts to the plan, you can expect to lose up to 10 pounds a month, or roughly 2 pounds every week. You may find that the number of inches you shave from your measurements makes it seem like 5 pounds a week.

It works. It's effective, and perhaps most important, it's delicious. Are you still a little worried about how all of this—particularly with the focus on fat—is going to affect your health? Then turn the page. We have the studies and information you need to ease your worried mind.

LOSE WEIGHT, GET HEALTHY, FEEL BETTER

Are you planning to try this diet, lose some weight, and then go back to some other "healthier" way of eating? We don't blame you for having this view. In fact, many years ago Valerie—like most nutritionists at the time—shared this view. That changed when she counseled a series of patients who were not only losing weight by consuming large amounts of fat, but who were also getting healthier. She watched as they started burning fat instead of storing it—and as their blood insulin, blood sugar, blood pressure, and cholesterol levels improved.

It changed everything. It revolutionized her thinking about nutrition. And it set her on the path that led to the groundbreaking work we've done at the Center for Balanced Health. We've seen our approach work on thousands of patients, people who'd all but given up hope of ever losing weight, or getting off medication, or having a child. We're pretty confident that, if you take the time to read the following pages carefully and with an open mind, it will transform the way you think about healthy nutrition, too. You see, the scientific evidence, studies, and testimonials all lead to one conclusion: When combined with high fiber intake, our high-fat approach not only enables weight loss without hunger, but it also helps reduce your risk for heart disease, cancer, stroke, diabetes, polycystic ovarian syndrome, osteoporosis, and overall aging. It also improves sleep, energy levels, and GI health.

Surprised? We bet you are, as most major media outlets have quoted so-called experts waxing poetic about the potential diseases that could be caused by eating too much fat. Yet such claims are without merit.

We, by the way, have the studies. Based on our experiences with thousands of patients and based on dozens of highly respected research papers published in peer-reviewed journals such as the *Journal of the American Medical Association* and the *Journal of Nutrition Research*, we can tell you with conviction that the high-fat diet we recommend will not shorten your life. It will not give you a heart attack. It will not raise your risk for cancer. If you follow the diet we recommend, you will:

- Stabilize your blood sugar and blood insulin levels, reducing your risk for polycystic ovarian syndrome, diabetes, and dangerously low blood sugar.
- Reduce cholesterol, blood pressure, and other heart disease risk factors.
- Lower your risk for cancer.
- Improve GI health and immunity by controlling yeast and promoting optimal bacteria balance in the intestinal tract.
- Improve thyroid and adrenal health, and, in turn, improve energy levels and mood, too.
- Strengthen your bones.
- Lose stubborn weight.
- Add years and quality to your life.

Yes, you will. You really will. We know it's hard to believe. We know it goes against everything you've been taught for the past 20 years, but read on. Keep your mind open. By the end of this Chapter, we're quite confident that you'll realize that everything you've been told about fat has been a big fat lie.

EAT FAT, LIVE LONGER

You've probably heard that the typical American diet—with its high emphasis on fatty cuts of meat—is what causes heart disease. We're wondering, however, if anyone ever told you about the high-fat diets of the Masai? No, you say? That's the answer we expected you to give, because many industry groups would probably rather you didn't know about the Masai and others who seem to thrive on a high-fat diet. It seems to confuse the low-fat message, doesn't it?

The Masai are a tribe in Africa that consumes a diet that is almost 100 percent saturated fat. Whole milk and beef are dietary staples. Do the

FAT: THE WHOLE TRUTH

Besides improving the taste and texture of food, dietary fat is vitally important for good health. Dietary fat:

- Is critical for proper brain and nerve function, eyesight, skin health, and even sperm count.
- Slows the progression of age-related memory loss and other cognitive disorders.
- Bolsters mood and prevents depression.
- Is used to make cell membranes, hormones, and hormonelike substances.
- Carries the fat-soluble vitamins A, D, E, and K. (Without fat, you'd become deficient in these vitamins.)
- Helps convert carotenes into vitamin A.
- Enables mineral absorption.
- Allows the body to fill in bone with calcium and other minerals.

Masai drop dead from heart attacks at age 40? No, they do not. The members of this tribe do not suffer from heart disease. They just don't get it.

Are they genetic anomalies? Do they lack a heart disease gene? It's not likely.

The Masai are just one of many societies around the globe that thrives on a diet rich in fat. The Inuit are another example. They live in North America and also develop little to no heart disease, obesity, and diabetes. They also eat a considerable amount of saturated fat, mostly from whales, fish, seals, and other animals. Is it possible that the Inuit, like the Masai, lack the heart disease and diabetes genes? It's possible, but not likely. You want to know why? Canadian Arctic explorer Vilhjalmur Stefansson lived with the Inuit for a year and consumed their fatty diet. He suffered no ill health effects.

How can this be? How can so many populations from so many different places in the world consume diets rich in animal fat and manage to stay healthy? They can because animal fat alone is not what causes heart disease, cancer, and other health problems. It's not until members of these healthy-fat-eating societies start eating typical American convenience foods such as fast food and processed foods that their rates of heart disease start to climb. It appears that natural sources of fat are not what make Americans more likely to suffer a heart attack than folks living in other countries around the world. It's the sugar, processed flour and starch, and synthetic fats.

Indeed, consider that a recent Harvard study followed the eating habits and health outcomes of more than 80,000 nurses over 2 decades. Women who consumed higher amounts of carbohydrates from refined sugar and highly processed foods nearly doubled their risk of heart disease compared to women who ate a lower carbohydrate diet. This latter group actually cut their risk of heart disease by 30 percent on average. At least five other studies—conducted at prestigious institutions such as Duke University and the University of Pennsylvania—show similar results for heart disease risk reduction.

Finally, a 2-year study that compared a high-fat, low-carb diet similar to ours to a low-fat diet and the Mediterranean diet (which emphasizes poultry, fish, olive oil, and nuts) determined that the low-carb dieters lost nearly twice as much weight as the low-fat dieters. And they were healthier at the end of the study. Their cholesterol profiles improved the most.

THE BIG FAT LIE

Are you feeling a little uneasy about what we've told you so far? Does it go against everything you've read, been taught, or believe about basic nutrition? We bet it does! We've counseled patient after patient who, after we suggested eating more fat and less carbohydrate, said something to the effect of, "What, are you trying to kill me?"

We're not.

Our patients and clients have also confessed to us, "My doctor gave me the okay to follow your diet and suggested I go off the diet as soon as I lose the weight." We're not sure of the rationale, but this advice seems more than just a little impractical. If a person loses weight and improves health, why in the world would you tell him or her to go back to eating the same foods that caused their health problems in the first place?

Think about it this way. This is a healthy nutrition plan filled with "clean foods," very little commercially prepared food, lots of vegetables, and moderate amounts of protein and fat (from natural sources such as nuts, avocados, seeds, olives, and meat). It is the plan that we recommend not only to our patients but also to friends and family. Neither of us needs to lose weight these days, but we both follow the approach laid out in this book, and we have done so for years. Would we do that if we thought it was going to kill us? Would we have our three children eating the same diet if we thought it would harm them? Would we recommend it to our patients, friends, and families if we thought there was any harm in eating this way?

No, no, and no.

We're trying to help you not only lose weight, but also live longer and, most important, love living. If we wanted to shorten your life span, we'd recommend the diet that so many of our colleagues are recommending these days. We'd tell you to start the day with breakfast cereal, have a sandwich and pretzels for lunch, and finish the day with pasta for dinner. If you feel hungry between meals, reach for a low-fat snack such as rice cakes, yogurt, crackers, or snack chips.

For most people, that's a recipe for a short life!

Once you have tried our diet, seen your health improve, and made strides toward your goals, we're pretty sure you'll come to the same conclusion and feel just as committed to this way of eating as we do. Right now, however, we know how it is. You need some convincing. You're probably feeling a little unsure of what to believe right now, and for good reason. You've been conditioned to fear fat. Valerie herself was a vegetarian who previously followed a low-fat diet—and she's a registered dietitian who was educated on all the principles that would contradict the very philosophy that she now advocates.

If she's had a change of heart about fat, you can rest assured that it only came after much scientific study, personal observation, and practical experience. She didn't change her mind on the topic overnight.

So, if it's a lie that fat is bad for our health, who started the lie? It was a researcher by the name of Ancel Keys. When studying the diets of various cultures around the world during the 1950s, Keys noticed that American business executives, who tended to eat a lot of fat, suffered greatly from heart disease. He also noticed that heart disease rates had dropped in post-war Europe as people were forced to survive on little food. He went on to study the diets and rates of heart disease in many additional countries, and in 1953 he published the "Seven Countries Study." In it, he concluded that dietary fat caused the high blood cholesterol levels that led to heart disease. It's Key's study from the 1950s that spurred the low-fat eating trend, not to mention many years and hundreds of millions of research dollars invested in additional studies that attempted to prove a connection between eating fat and having a heart attack.

You know what? No additional studies were able to prove a link between dietary fat, cholesterol levels, and heart disease. To the contrary, studies show the opposite.

The lack of evidence for the low-fat diet did not stop the United States and other governments from turning Key's initial findings into dogma. In January 1977, a Senate committee led by George McGovern published its "Dietary Goals for the United States," advising Americans to cut back on fat. In 1984 the National Institutes of Health recommended that all Americans older than age 2 rein in fat. The nation's top health organizations, including the American Heart Association, cling to this dietary advice, despite lots of evidence that shows it may do more harm than good.

THE AMERICAN PARADOX

Before the 1920s, heart disease was rare in the United States. By the mid 1950s, however, heart disease was the leading cause of death, as it still is today, for both men and women.

If fat is so bad for us, one would assume that Americans started eating more of it in the 1900s, in step with these rising rates of heart disease, not to mention rising rates of diabetes and obesity. That assumption, however, is incorrect.

Internationally renowned nutritionist and biochemist Mary G. Enig, PhD, has studied the eating patterns of Americans dating back as far as the late 1800s. In her highly regarded book *Know Your Fats* (Bethesda Press, 2000), she convincingly uses U.S. Department of Agriculture data to show that fat consumption and heart disease have no connection whatsoever. According to her review of government health records and food consumption statistics, Americans cut back on animal fat between 1910 and 1970. In the early 1900s, Americans were eating mostly saturated and monounsaturated fats in the form of butter, lard, coconut oil, and olive oil. By the 1970s, Americans were eating fewer animal fats and less butter and lard. Since the 1970s, Americans have cut back on saturated fat even more.

Has all of this fat cutting done any good for our hearts? No. Heart disease rates are going up, not down.

If it's not animal fat, then what is clogging our arteries and trigger-

Nadine E. **Normalized Her Blood Sugar and Controlled Her Diabetes!**

I was diagnosed with type 2 diabetes in 1997 and have since been taking a number of medications to control my blood sugar.

The first 2 days of the diet were tough but I followed it strictly for 2 weeks. I found myself looking for carbs. I was used to grabbing foods off my children's plates. Valerie helped me to be more aware of what I was reaching for and why. Then my body got used to it and I got used to it, and the cravings diminished.

The biggest change for me was breakfast. I had been eating oatmeal, but I switched to eggs. I also learned to have a low-carbohydrate snack either just before or during my children's snack times, so I would not be tempted to nibble on whatever they were having.

It's a healthy way of eating. I am eating real foods rather than processed foods. I am eating fruit, vegetables, and protein foods—all foods that are good for you. Occasionally, I'll indulge in 70 percent chocolate. When I eat starch, like pasta or brown rice, I eat only one serving so that my blood sugar remains in control. Once in a blue moon I might have a sugar-free ice cream, but that's it. I might have a bite of a higher-carbohydrate food from time to time, but I don't eat a whole serving. These small treats are what make the plan livable.

I had unbelievable results. In just 6 weeks I not only lost 6 pounds, but my blood glucose normalized. My blood glucose dropped from 92 to 89, and my HbA1c was 5.8 percent! I was able to stop taking *all* of my medicines. I'm technically not diabetic anymore. I feel good, really good, and I'm so happy to not be taking my prescriptions.

ing heart attacks in record numbers? The answer to that question points to at least three additives and food ingredients: refined flour, added sugar and high-fructose corn syrup, and synthetic "partially hydrogenated" fats (also called trans fats). During the past 100 years and particularly since the 1970s, Americans have consumed all three in record amounts, and we have the hearts to show for it.

THE DANGERS OF FAKE FAT

Trans fatty acids are created when manufacturers partially hydrogenate vegetable oils, whipping the fats with hydrogen to make them solid at room temperature. These fats were invented in a lab a century ago to provide a cheap alternative to butter. At the time, it may have seemed like a good idea, but maybe the joke is on us. The consumption of hydrogenated trans fats from vegetable oils (found in margarine, baked goods, fried foods, and most processed foods) jumped 400 percent during the 1900s.

Consider:

- An 8-year Harvard study of more than 18,000 women determined that each 2 percent increase in the consumption of trans fats resulted in a 73 percent greater risk of infertility and ovulation problems. Other types of fat, however, did not raise the risk of infertility.
- In Harvard's ongoing Nurses Health Study, women with the highest amounts of trans fats in their blood cells were three times as likely to develop heart disease compared to women with the lowest levels.
- In a 10-year Harvard study of more than 16,000 men, each 2 percent increase in trans fats consumption (substituted for either another type of fat or carbohydrates) resulted in a 0.30 inch increase in waist circumference.

Studies have linked trans fats with an increased risk of heart disease, cancer, diabetes, immunity, reproductive problems, and obesity.

THE IMPORTANCE OF FAT BALANCE

The consumption of trans fats, sugar, and refined carbohydrates may not be the only factor in the rising rates of heart disease in this country. An imbalance in our consumption of different types of fat may also contribute to the problem. As it turns out, our bodies evolved on a diet that was relatively rich in a type of fat called omega-3 fatty acids (found in salmon and walnuts, among other foods) and relatively low in omega-6 fatty acids (found in many vegetable oils, particularly soy and corn oil). Many researchers believe that no more than twice as many fat calories should come from omega-6 fats as from omega-3 fats, but most of us are consuming 25 *times* as much omega-6 fats as omega-3s.

Our consumption of omega-3s are low for a number of reasons. Few of us eat enough fatty fish, walnuts, flax, greens, and other foods that are rich in this type of fat. Commercial farming also reduces the natural omega-3 fats that would normally be present in animal meat, eggs, and vegetables.

THE TRUE CORONARY CULPRITS

Countries that consume diets rich in saturated fat tend to suffer very little heart disease, whereas countries that consume diets rich in hydrogenated trans fats suffer high rates of heart disease. Population studies show that people who eat small amounts of trans fats, white flour, or sugar do not have heart attacks. Common sense should tell us that the problem isn't animal fat alone. It's trans fats, sugar, high-fructose corn syrup, and refined carbohydrates.

Eggs from hens that eat insects and green plants, for example, are richer in omega-3s than eggs from hens that are fed soy. Worse, most processed foods are loaded with omega-6 fats from corn or soybean oil.

This imbalance of omega-3s to omega-6s throws off our delicate metabolic balance, triggering the body to make more pro-inflammatory substances that raise blood pressure, irritate the GI tract, lower immunity, and even contribute to weight gain. This contributes to cancer, heart disease, poor immunity, liver damage, reproductive problems, GI distress, learning disabilities, and overweight.

WHAT REALLY RAISES CHOLESTEROL

You might still be scratching your head, thinking to yourself, "I know I've heard about studies that prove that saturated fat raises cholesterol."

You heard correctly. Saturated fat does tend to raise total cholesterol, but that may not necessarily raise your risk of heart disease. This is where things get a little complicated, so please bear with us. As it turns out, cholesterol is more complicated than one number. Years ago, we were told to keep total cholesterol under 200 mg/dl. Today, we know that total cholesterol matters much less than the types of cholesterol in the blood. If you have high total cholesterol, but most of it is the good HDL type, your risk of heart disease is probably lower than that of someone who has seemingly normal total cholesterol, but low HDL.

When it comes to cholesterol, here's what matters and why.

LDL cholesterol. Known as the "bad" cholesterol, LDL has been thought to come to rest along the linings of arteries, get stuck, and build up into plaque. As it turns out, there are at least two types of LDL particles—small and large. If more than 22 percent of your LDL is the small, dense type, your risk of developing heart disease is three times higher than if you have larger LDL particles, even if your total LDL is considered normal. Research from the University of California at Berkeley has determined that people with larger LDL particles in their blood either get no benefit from low-fat diets or they experience an increased risk of heart disease as their LDL particles switch from large to small in size. When you replace carbohydrate with fat, dangerous small LDL particles tend to get bigger, so your risk goes down.

Apoliprotein B (also called Apo B). Part of LDL cholesterol, Apo B in high levels has been linked to heart disease. Research at Children's Hospital Oakland Research Institute in California shows that Apo B rises when study participants switch to a low-fat, high-carbohydrate diet.

HDL cholesterol. For many years HDL has been considered the "good" cholesterol because it tends to carry fat back to the liver rather than get stuck in the artery lining. Recent research, however, has shown that, like LDL, there may be many types of HDL, some more desirable than others. In a study published in the *American Journal of Clinical Nutrition*, participants who restricted carbohydrates improved their HDL levels twice as much as participants who restricted fat. Other research shows that low-fat, high-carbohydrate diets tend to lower HDL, increasing your risk for heart disease.

Triglycerides. This fat is stored in fat cells and circulated in the blood to provide fuel for cells. Levels tend to rise after a meal, as the body sends excess calories, in the form of triglycerides, to fat cells for storage. You might think that a diet rich in fat would cause these blood fats to jump. It doesn't necessarily, assuming you pair your high-fat intake with a low intake of carbohydrates.

When you consume a low-carbohydrate, high-fat diet, your body burns triglycerides for fuel, so levels drop rather than go up, and your body burns fat rather than stores it. Eating a diet low in fat and high in carbohydrates does the opposite by converting excess carbohydrates into triglycerides and eventually storing them as fat. In fact, 85 percent of excess carbs are converted into triglycerides. Excess carbohydrates that can't be immediately used for energy or stored in your muscles as glycogen go back to the liver, where they're converted into triglycerides and circulate in your blood until they come to rest either inside a fat cell or along the sides of your arteries.

C-Reactive Protein (CRP). High levels of this inflammatory marker raise your risk for heart disease. Weight loss tends to improve CRP levels.

So, you see, our bodies were designed to consume animal and vegetable fats. In fact, certain types of fat, such as the unsaturated fat found
in olive oil, are good for you, raising levels of the good HDL cholesterol and lowering levels of the bad LDL cholesterol. These foods also
contain important nutrients that are important for heart health. For
example, the folic acid in avocados helps improve heart health. Saturated fat, found in meat and eggs, is neutral; it raises levels of both types
of cholesterol. As Harvard researchers have discovered, you damage
your heart health much more by forgoing these healthy fats in favor of
processed carbohydrates.

WHY INSULIN MATTERS THE MOST

Your insulin level probably matters much more to your overall health
than your cholesterol level does. Whereas high levels of certain types of
cholesterol have been linked with heart disease, high insulin levels have
been linked with nearly every health-related cause of death. High insulin levels have been associated with obesity, heart disease, diabetes,
cancer, and overall aging. A low-carbohydrate diet drives down insulin, whereas a high-carbohydrate diet raises it.

Here's how high insulin levels can increase your risk for a number
of diseases.

Heart disease. High insulin levels trigger the liver to produce triglycerides, raising your risk for heart disease. In the 22-year Helsinki
Finnish Policeman study of 970 men, the men with the highest insulin
levels were most likely to suffer a heart attack over the course of the
study. Other studies have yielded similar results.

Reduced life span. Researchers have long known that people who
reduce their insulin levels either through exercise or calorie restriction tend
to live longer than people with higher insulin levels. For example, studies
show that centenarians tend to have lower insulin levels than people who
die earlier, and their cells tend to be more sensitive to the hormone's effects.
High insulin levels have been shown to speed the aging rate of cells and
tissues throughout the body. When insulin levels remain low, cells more
easily fight off age-related diseases such as cancer, dementia, and stroke.

High blood pressure. If your cells are resistant to insulin and,
consequently, insulin levels rise, this causes the body to excrete magnesium. Cells need magnesium to relax. When levels are low, blood
vessels constrict and blood pressure rises.

AS CLEAR AS THE NOSE ON YOUR FACE

When 50 teenage boys in an Australian study stopped eating junk foods laden with sugar and high-fructose corn syrup, their acne cleared up. The results were better than those of over-the-counter acne medications. The low-sugar diet works, yet again, by reducing insulin levels and normalizing levels of other key hormones.

Weak bones. Insulin affects other hormones such as growth hormone, testosterone, and progesterone. When cells become resistant to insulin and levels rise, bone-building hormonal signals get distorted, causing the body to excrete calcium and weaken bones.

What raises insulin? In a word: excess carbohydrates, especially from sugar and refined grains. When you consume grains and starches, the pancreas must produce insulin, with high-glycemic, faster-digesting carbs creating a greater and more rapid response than lower-glycemic carbs. Individually, fat and fiber do not trigger a response.

WHAT ABOUT CANCER?

Have you read or heard that diets high in fat raise your risk of developing certain cancers, especially breast cancer and colon cancer? A number of studies have come to these conclusions and seem to support the message that dietary fat is bad for your health.

At first glance, such research certainly seems damning, but there are at least two huge problems with many of the studies that have linked high-fat diets with cancer.

1. **The people who consumed high amounts of fat, in these studies, also consumed low amounts of vegetables.** The typical American diet is also very low in vegetables, with most people consuming one or fewer servings a day. Vegetables are a rich source of antioxidants, nutrients that are important in preventing the DNA damage that can lead to cancer. They also tend to be alkalinizing to the body, balancing body pH, which also improves health.

2. **The people who consumed high amounts of fat tended to consume this fat from foods that contain known carcinogens,** such as lunch meat and bacon, both of which contains nitrates.

We are not aware of any studies that have linked a healthy, high-fat diet with increased cancer risk. The studies that have been done have not controlled for meats containing nitrates and meats that do not contain known carcinogens. The research has been done on the typical American diet, which is not only high in fat but also high in sugar, processed foods, cured lunch meats, pesticide residues, food contaminants, and many other carcinogens.

More carefully designed studies show the opposite: Fat does *not* raise cancer risk. Consider:

- A study of women in early-stage breast cancer tracked the outcomes of one group who consumed low-fat diets rich in vegetables, fruits, and fiber and another group who ate five or more servings of vegetables or fruit a day without restricting fat. The women in the low-fat group had the same risk of cancer recurrence as did women in the high-fat group, showing that fat isn't the issue. More likely, lack of vegetables is.
- A 20-year Harvard study of more than 80,000 women found that high waist circumference (an "apple" body shape) raised risk for breast cancer, but a high-fat diet did not. In fact, women with insulin resistance who consumed a high-fat diet experienced a drop in breast cancer risk.
- A Harvard review of 12 studies involving more than 500,000 women concluded that neither total fat nor type of fat influenced the risk of developing ovarian cancer.
- The same holds true for pancreatic cancer and colon cancer.

What *does* cause cancer? We were hoping you'd ask. As it turns out, an unbalanced diet that includes too many carbohydrates—especially from sugar and processed starch—has been shown to be a main contributor. In yet another Harvard study of more than 1,700 women, those who consumed more carbohydrates, especially from sweeteners such as sugar and high-fructose corn syrup, were more likely to develop breast cancer than women who consumed fewer carbohydrates. Healthy cells can make energy from fat and from ketones (a by-product of fat burning) and do not need sugar to maintain health. Cancer cells need sugar to grow and divide. A number of researchers around the globe are experimenting with carbohydrate-free diets (known as the ketogenic diet) to see whether they can cure cancer. Results have been encouraging. For example, five patients in Germany who had been diagnosed with late-stage terminal cancers either stabilized or improved after 3 months of a near-zero-carbohydrate diet. Their tumors either stopped growing or shrunk! (The ketogenic diet, by the way, has been used for years to reduce seizures in children with epilepsy.)

Also, it's processed vegetable oil, not animal fat, that may cause cancer. Research by Mary G. Enig, PhD, completed during a 60-year period, determined that cancer rates rose when people consumed hydrogenated vegetable oils (trans fats), and not when people consumed saturated fats. According to Enig's research, the increased consumption of trans fats correlated with increasing cancer rates.

For these reasons and more, the diet we promote is rich in healthy fats, vegetables, and fiber. Remember: It's all about balance. You can eat as many vegetables as you want—even the ones that have fat in them—and you'll never consume enough vegetable oil to throw your body out of balance. It's when you overconsume vegetable oil in the form of cooking oil or as soybean and other types of oil in just about every processed food that problems result. Vegetables are good. Processed oil from vegetables isn't.

GOOD FOR LIFE

By now, we hope we've convinced you that this diet—with its emphasis on health-promoting natural foods—not only is safe for weight loss but also is loaded with nutrients so that you can enjoy eating this way for the rest of your life. It's a healthful diet for men and women of every age—and even for children.

It's healthy. It's effective. It's delicious.

Are you ready to dig in and try it? Then turn to Chapter 5 to learn more about your metabolism, and how it affects the best food choices and supplements for you.

FAT FIGHTS FREE RADICALS

Diets high in fat and very low in carbohydrates have been shown to enhance the body's ability to fight free radicals, substances thought to lead to heart disease, cancer, and premature aging.

FAT 101

Here's a rundown of the different types of fat and how they affect cholesterol.

Monounsaturated fats. Found in olives and olive oil; avocados; peanuts and most other nuts; and many seeds, including pumpkin and flaxseeds or flax oil, these fats are relatively good for you. They tend to raise your good HDL cholesterol and lower your bad LDL cholesterol.

Polyunsaturated fats. These fats are found in plant oils, and some types decrease both LDL and HDL. There are many types of polyunsaturated fats, including omega-3 fats, omega-6 fats, and omega-9 fats. Of these, omega-3s are most beneficial to heart health—they've been shown to lower triglycerides and blood pressure and prevent blood clots. They are found in salmon, mackerel, herring, halibut, scallops, and shrimp. Plant foods such as flaxseeds and walnuts contain a type of fat called alpha-linolenic acid that is converted into the usable form of omega-3 by the body. Other sources of omega-3s are dark green vegetables such as seaweed, broccoli, spinach, and kale. It's thought that consuming a diet high in omega-6 fats (found in vegetable oils, such as corn and soy) and low in omega-3 fats increases the risk of heart disease.

Saturated fats. Found in animal products, there are many types of saturated fat. Some have no effect on cholesterol (stearic acid), whereas others raise bad (LDL) cholesterol. Most raise both LDL and HDL, making them heart disease neutral.

Trans fats. These come mostly from partially hydrogenated vegetable oils in restaurant fryers, margarines, packaged snacks, and baked goods. These fats raise the risk of heart disease by upping the bad LDL cholesterol and triglycerides and lowering the good HDL cholesterol. Although they occur in small amounts in meat, they primarily come from packaged baked products (cookies, cakes, breads, crackers) and fast food. Eat as few trans fats as possible. They are listed on labels, but be careful of packaging. A food can claim that it contains zero trans fats even if it has 0.5 gram or less. If you eat more than a single portion, you may be getting more trans fats than you bargained for.

PICK YOUR PLAN

We're thrilled that you've decided to embark on the program. We're quite confident that you will not be disappointed.

We'd like to start you on your road to weight loss in the same way we start all of our patients. We'd like to get to know you better. If you can get to Manhattan, we suggest you come to our medical practice for a physical exam, blood work, and some face time. This book, however, is the next best thing to a visit and will give you a broad scope of information that will help you live healthier and slim for the rest of your life.

We're with you, so let's get started. If you have a medical condition that warrants professional care, however, this book is not a substitute for human care. Continue to consult with your health care provider to ensure that you receive the best care for your current situation.

The following reflective questions and self-assessments will help you determine important personality traits, physical symptoms, and lifestyle habits that affect how you should eat, which supplements you should take, and when and how much you should exercise. Your results will also determine which of the two eating programs you should begin with. You see, no single eating plan fits all people. If you've ever been on a diet before, you know this!

DO YOU HAVE A METABOLIC DISADVANTAGE?

The vast majority of people who are overweight—especially people who have struggled unsuccessfully to lose weight—generally have a metabolic problem that is working against them. Without the right supplements, fiber, and nutrient-rich vegetables, plus a strict avoidance of certain types of both carbohydrates and fats for an extended period of time, these metabolic problems do not resolve. To enable weight loss, you must fix the problem, and, to fix the problem, you must know one exists in the first place.

To determine whether you have one or more metabolic disadvantages, answer the following questions in each category.

Insulin Disadvantage

Answer each of the following questions with a yes or no.

1. Do commercially prepared carbohydrate foods (such as bread, cereal, pasta, potatoes, rice, beans, desserts, soft drinks, and fruit) make up more than 40 percent of each meal or snack that you eat?

    ☐ YES   ☐ NO

2. Between meals, do you feel hungry or crave sweets, starches (such as bread), or caffeine (such as coffee)?

    ☐ YES   ☐ NO

3. Do you feel as if you might be addicted to certain types of sweet foods—as if once you start eating these foods, you can't stop? When you eat them, do you feel high, followed quickly by an emotional low? ★★ (See page 76.)

    ☐ YES   ☐ NO

4. Have you at any time experienced any of the following: ★★

    ☐ Feeling thirstier than usual, despite normal water consumption

    ☐ Weight gain despite following a weight loss plan or trying to reduce calories or portions

    ☐ Sensation of your heart beating quickly (palpitations), even though you have not exerted yourself

    ☐ Feeling tired in the morning or during the day, despite adequate sleep

    ☐ Feeling sleepy or drowsy after meals

    ☐ Feeling shaky when you are hungry

☐ Feeling faint if you delay a meal or snack by 30 to 60 minutes

☐ Trembling (shaking) of the hands

☐ Blurred vision

☐ Bleeding gums, despite good dental care

☐ A tingling sensation in your legs or feet

☐ Low sex drive/libido (lower than in the past or than what you'd like)

☐ Impotence or erectile dysfunction

☐ Muscle twitching or cramps

☐ Excessive sweating, even if you have not exerted yourself

☐ Fatigue that is relieved by eating

☐ Dizziness, giddiness, or lightheadedness

5. Have you noticed a change in your ability to focus or concentrate?

☐ YES   ☐ NO

6. Have you recently developed headaches, suffering one more than once a week?

☐ YES   ☐ NO

7. Do you feel you have a diminished ability to work under pressure?

☐ YES   ☐ NO

8. Do you get up to urinate at night? ★★

☐ YES   ☐ NO

9. Do you frequently wake before 5 a.m., even though you have not set an alarm? ★★

☐ YES   ☐ NO

10. Do you wake feeling hungry, dry mouthed, or dehydrated? ★★

☐ YES   ☐ NO

(continued on page 76)

11. Do you gain weight in your stomach rather than in your hips or thighs?

☐ YES   ☐ NO

Your number of "yes" answers: _____

If you answered yes to two or more questions, you probably have an insulin disadvantage. Consider making an appointment with your primary care physician. Mention that you think you may have an insulin or blood sugar disorder, and be sure to say whether or not this problem runs in your family. Explain that you are interested in a glucose tolerance test. If you have hypoglycemia (low blood sugar, an early warning sign that diabetes is developing), your 90-minute glucose reading will be lower than your fasting glucose reading. You also might experience a drop in glucose of greater than 30 mm in an hour, or your reading may be below 70. Your sugar is overly high if your fasting glucose is greater than 100, your 2-hour glucose is greater than 140, or if at any point during the test your glucose rises above 200. If you test normal on your blood work but you answered yes to any of the starred questions in the quiz, you may be developing an insulin disadvantage that is not yet extreme enough to be detected. If you make no changes to your lifestyle, it may eventually show up!

If you have an insulin disadvantage, you must strictly adhere to Level 1 eating and you will probably have to stay at this level for a longer period of time than someone who does not have an insulin disadvantage. We recommend you follow Level 1 for at least a month, deviating only as needed to ensure that you don't lose momentum and stop following the plan altogether. You'll find specific advice for how to modify the plan for success in Chapters 6 and 12. You also need additional supplements, outlined in Chapter 9.

Yeast Disadvantage

Answer each of the following questions with a yes or no.

1. Do you experience gas, especially after eating sugar, foods than contain vinegar, cured foods, pickled foods, sun-dried tomatoes, moldy cheeses (i.e. blue cheese), and mushrooms? ★★

☐ YES   ☐ NO

2. Does your abdomen fill up with air (bloating) after you eat, at night, or periodically throughout the day? ★★

☐ YES   ☐ NO

3. Have you been diagnosed with ulcers, gastritis, or irritable bowel syndrome? ★★

☐ YES   ☐ NO

4. Do you frequently experience indigestion or a "nervous stomach"? ★★

☐ YES   ☐ NO

5. Is diarrhea or constipation a daily concern? ★★

☐ YES   ☐ NO

6. Do you regularly experience brain fog (the sensation that you can't concentrate or think clearly), despite adequate sleep?

☐ YES   ☐ NO

7. Is your lack of focus affecting your ability to accomplish minor tasks?

☐ YES   ☐ NO

8. Have you been sick frequently or taken antibiotics more than three times in a year?

☐ YES   ☐ NO

9. Do you ever develop hives, acne, or rosacea?

☐ YES   ☐ NO

10. Does your tongue have a white coating?

☐ YES   ☐ NO

11. Do you have seasonal allergies, food allergies, or allergies to medications?

☐ YES   ☐ NO

12. Are your sinuses frequently stuffy or infected?

☐ YES   ☐ NO

13. Do you have asthma?

☐ YES   ☐ NO

14. Have you been diagnosed with an ulcer or gastric reflux?

☐ YES   ☐ NO

Your number of "yes" answers: _____

If you have a normal test result but answered yes to two or more questions, you may have a yeast disadvantage. This means you have an overgrowth of yeast or unhealthy bacteria (or both) in your digestive tract. Consider making an appointment with your physician. If you have a normal test result but answered yes to any of the starred questions in the quiz, you may be developing a yeast disadvantage that is not yet extreme enough to be detected by medical tests. If you make no changes to your lifestyle, it may eventually show up.

If you have just 5 to 10 pounds to lose, use the Level 2 eating plan until you reach your goal. If you have more weight to lose, use Level 1. Regardless of the plan, for 3 to 6 months you should avoid the following yeast-promoting foods: fermented, pickled, and moldy (blue cheese) foods; soy sauce; vinegar; mushrooms; sour cream; sauerkraut; some nuts (cashews, peanuts, pistachios); pickles; breads that contain yeast; and all cheese except mozzarella and cream cheese. It's also particularly important for you to maximize your 3 to 7 cups of green leafy vegetables and 2 cups of other vegetables every day. Vegetables contain fiber, and fiber nourishes the healthy bacteria in your digestive tract. Finally, you will need to take additional supplements, outlined in Chapter 9.

Thyroid Disadvantage

Answer each of the following questions with a yes or no.

1. Do you suffer from cold hands and feet, even when you are in a heated room? ★★

        ☐ YES   ☐ NO

2. Do you feel depressed, lethargic, unmotivated, or hopeless?

        ☐ YES   ☐ NO

3. Do you suffer from constipation?

        ☐ YES   ☐ NO

4. Do your nails break easily?

        ☐ YES   ☐ NO

5. Do you have a low sex drive/libido (lower than in the past or than what you'd like)?

        ☐ YES   ☐ NO

6. Do you have difficulty sleeping (it takes you longer than 30 minutes to fall asleep and you wake more than once at night)?

☐ YES ☐ NO

7. Do you feel tired during the day?

☐ YES ☐ NO

8. Have you recently gained weight, even though you were not overeating? ★★

☐ YES ☐ NO

9. Have the hairs along the outer one-third of your eyebrows thinned or fallen out? ★★

☐ YES ☐ NO

10. Do you suffer from muscle aches or joint pain, despite doing nothing more rigorous than your daily activities?

☐ YES ☐ NO

11. Is your temperature below 98.5°F when you first wake up? ★★

☐ YES ☐ NO

12. Is your total cholesterol above 200 or your LDL cholesterol above 130?

☐ YES ☐ NO

Women Only:

1. Do you skip periods, have periods more frequently than once a month, or menstruate irregularly, even though you are not perimenopausal or postmenopausal?

☐ YES ☐ NO

2. Is your hair thinning?

☐ YES ☐ NO

Your number of "yes" answers: _____

If you answered yes to two or more questions, consider making an appointment with your physician for a thyroid test. If you have a normal test result but answered yes to any of the starred questions, you may have a thyroid issue that is too mild to be diagnosed by a medical test.

Follow the Level 2 eating plan and take the supplements outlined for the thyroid disadvantage in Chapter 9. You may not lose weight as quickly as someone who does not have a thyroid disadvantage, but you will see results and you can meet your goals.

Hormone Disadvantage

Answer each of the following questions with a yes or no.

1. Are you tired during the day?

☐ YES   ☐ NO

2. Do you have a low sex drive/libido (lower than in the past or than what you'd like)?

☐ YES   ☐ NO

3. Do you have difficulty sleeping (it takes you longer than 30 minutes to fall asleep, and you wake more than once at night)?

☐ YES   ☐ NO

4. Have you gained weight, despite following a weight loss plan or trying to reduce calories or portions?

☐ YES   ☐ NO

5. Are you depressed?

☐ YES   ☐ NO

Women only:

1. Is your hair thinning?

☐ YES   ☐ NO

2. Do you have facial hair?

☐ YES   ☐ NO

3. Do you retain water?

☐ YES   ☐ NO

4. Do you skip periods, have periods more frequently than once a month, or menstruate irregularly, even though you are not perimenopausal or postmenopausal? ★★

☐ YES   ☐ NO

5. Do you bleed heavily during your periods (soaking through a tampon or pad within an hour)? ★★

☐ YES   ☐ NO

6. Do you feel irritable, bloated, or fatigued in the days leading up to your period? ★★

☐ YES   ☐ NO

7. Do you have hot flashes or night sweats, even though you are not perimenopausal? ★★

☐ YES   ☐ NO

Men only:

1. Are you developing breasts? ★★

☐ YES   ☐ NO

2. Do you have impotence or erectile dysfunction? ★★

☐ YES   ☐ NO

3. Have you been diagnosed with a low sperm count? ★★

☐ YES   ☐ NO

Your number of "yes" answers: _____

If you found many of the hormone disadvantage questions similar to the thyroid questions, there's a good reason for that. These conditions generally overlap. Most people who have one condition also have the other. If you answered yes to two or more questions, consider making an appointment with your physician to test your testosterone levels (for men) and your estrogen and progesterone levels (for women). If you have a normal test result but answered yes to any of the starred questions in the quiz, you may be developing a hormone disadvantage that is not yet extreme enough to be detected by medical tests. If you make no changes to your lifestyle, it may eventually show up.

If despite a normal test result you suspect you may have a hormone disadvantage, follow Level 1 eating but do not use the specific hormone disadvantage supplements. These supplements are effective when treating a problem, but they do pose some risks. We don't want you to take them unless you are definitely sure you need them.

With a confirmed hormone disadvantage, follow Level 1 eating and use the supplements described in Chapter 9. You may not lose weight as quickly as someone who does not have a hormone disadvantage, but you will see results and you can meet your goals.

Adrenal Disadvantage

Answer each of the following questions with a yes or no.

1. Do you have trouble slowing down at night? ★★
   ☐ YES   ☐ NO

2. Does it take longer than 30 minutes for you to fall asleep? ★★
   ☐ YES   ☐ NO

3. Do you frequently wake at night and find yourself unable to get back to sleep? ★★
   ☐ YES   ☐ NO

4. Do you watch TV or use a computer shortly before bed?
   ☐ YES   ☐ NO

5. Do you eat while working, watching TV, or sitting at the computer?
   ☐ YES   ☐ NO

6. Do you have trouble getting out of bed in the morning because you do not feel rested?
   ☐ YES   ☐ NO

7. Do you keep yourself going during the day by drinking or taking caffeine?
   ☐ YES   ☐ NO

Your number of "yes" answers: _____

If you answered yes to one or more questions, consider talking to your doctor about testing your cortisol levels. High cortisol levels indicate that your stress response is turned "on" all day long. Low cortisol indicates that your adrenals have burned out. If you have a normal test result but answered yes to any of the starred questions in the quiz, you may be developing an adrenal disadvantage that is not yet extreme enough to be detected by medical tests. If you make no changes to your lifestyle, it may eventually show up.

In either case, follow Level 2 eating, take the supplements described in Chapter 9, and pay particular attention to the stress-reduction advice in Chapter 10. Also, it's particularly important for you to avoid cardiovascular exercise during the first month of your weight loss plan. You may not lose weight as quickly as someone who does not have an adrenal disadvantage, but you will see results and you can meet your goals.

Depending on the type and severity of your disadvantage, you must:

Start with the right eating plan for your body. If you are overweight *and* have an insulin, yeast, or hormone disadvantage, Level 1 is the best place to start. (However, if you have a yeast disadvantage but are close to your ideal weight, start at Level 2. Check the BMI chart (page 249) to determine your ideal weight.) These conditions mean that you are either in metabolic inflation or full-scale depression. The Level 1 plan is designed to reverse the inflation by lowering levels of insulin and other key hormones.

Level 1 is also the best place to start if you are healthy (have no disadvantages) and want to lose weight fast. (We'll go over all the particulars of Level 1 starting on page 107.)

If you have a thyroid or adrenal disadvantage, you'll start with the Level 2 plan (a full description of Level 2 starts on page 127). These disadvantages mean that your body is in a state of metabolic overspending and needs rest more than anything else. The Level 1 plan may not work for you and would add unnecessary stress to your already overworked organs.

If you are completely addicted to carbs (you know who you are), you can start with Level 2 and slowly ease yourself into Level 1 eating when you feel more in control. Then stick with Level 1 for at least 2 weeks (or at least a month, if you have an insulin disadvantage) before returning to Level 2 again.

You can also start with Level 2 if your goal is to lose 10 pounds or less.

Take additional supplements to fix your underlying medical problem. We recommend an assortment of supplements for everyone, metabolic disadvantage or not. If you have a metabolic disadvantage, however, you may need to take a few additional supplements or higher doses than the basic supplement plan we prescribe. We'll cover all of this in Chapter 9.

Start exercising later rather than sooner. If you have an adrenal or a thyroid disadvantage, you need rest. Consider it doctor's orders not to exercise. Exercise will only further tax your body, hindering weight loss rather than helping it. We don't recommend you start exercising until you've lost 10 percent of your initial weight, have established good sleep habits, and feel well rested. If you have any of the other disadvantages, you can start exercising as soon as you feel ready. Know that dietary changes are much more effective, however. If you only have the time or energy to make one change, change how you eat. Once you feel comfortable with your eating plan, transition into the exercise plan. A main benefit of exercise is to help maintain weight loss.

KNOW THYSELF, HEAL THYSELF

Now you have the answers as to why you need to modify your eating, exercise, and supplement plans accordingly. We hope this quiz brings you one step closer to getting to know your body better. If you have a metabolic disadvantage, that's why you've had such a hard time losing weight in the past. Now that you understand the problem, you have the information you need to motivate yourself to succeed. It's one thing to lose weight to look better. It's quite another to do it for your health. We've found that our most successful and most highly motivated patients were the ones who made their weight loss goal their top priority and shed negative behaviors and emotions along with their unhealthy habits.

You're almost ready to begin the program. Just a few more steps, and you'll be on your way. First, set a date to start—preferably soon! Doing so will help focus your energies and mark a clear separation from your unhealthy eating patterns of the past.

BEFORE DAY 1

Successful weight loss requires preparation. Before you change even one meal, do the following:

Read this book from cover to cover. We know many of you will read the next chapter, put down the book, and then get to the business of losing weight as soon as possible. We don't want you to do that—not yet! Please finish the entire book first. Wanting to get started *right this second* is understandable, but reaching your weight loss goal takes a lot more than knowing what to eat. You might be able to lose

METABOLICALLY CHALLENGED: DISADVANTAGES THAT SET YOU APART FROM THE REST

If you have more than one of the previously described disadvantages, then things are a little complicated. Do not feel bad about this. Most of the people we treat are in a similar situation. Many of the metabolic disadvantages are interrelated. For example, most people with an insulin disadvantage also have an adrenal disadvantage. Most people with a thyroid disadvantage also have a hormone disadvantage (especially postmenopausal women). No matter how disadvantaged your metabolism, if you follow our eating plan, take the right supplements, and implement the stress-reducing advice outlined in Chapter 10, you will succeed! Just be patient, though, because you will not lose weight as quickly as someone who does not have these disadvantages. The weight will come off slowly, but it will come off. You'll probably shrink inches before you drop pounds, but eventually you will see lower numbers on the scale (and on your clothing tags).

weight for a while with no preparation and with no supportive information, but you'll eventually hit a rough patch. When you do, come back to the book. We've tried to include all of the advice that helps our clients and patients overcome barriers. It's all in here! No matter what your reasons for wanting to quit the program, come back to the book and see whether you can find a solution to the problem, or try to think of your own creative ways to overcome stumbling blocks.

Get a full checkup. If you're still worried about how this diet might affect your heart health, ask your primary care physician to run a full cholesterol and blood sugar panel. Follow up once every few months as you lose weight to ensure that these health indicators are all moving in the right direction.

Go shopping. Purchase the supplements you need (outlined in Chapter 9) and head to the grocery store for healthy lower-carb staples such as fresh and frozen vegetables, eggs, cocoa, cream, avocados, olives, coconut oil, and an assortment of meat and fish. Use the list on page 99 as a guide.

Rearrange your kitchen. Which types of food do you have sitting in plain view? Which foods will you see every time you open the refrigerator, freezer, or cupboard? Many clients have told us that they've easily gone days or weeks without pasta, potatoes, bread, or other high-carbohydrate foods, but when they saw those foods—say their spouse brought home a fresh crusty loaf of bread from the bakery—they lost their resolve. If possible, get rid of tempting foods that you will not be eating in the coming weeks. If other family members complain, put these foods in an inconvenient location or out of sight. For example, put bread in the freezer. Put snack chips in the highest kitchen cabinet, one you do not open very often. Put chocolate and other extremely tempting foods in an opaque container, and put the container out of sight, too.

Talk to your family. Explain that you will be embarking on a new way of eating and that you need their support. Explain why you want to lose weight. Be honest. Talk about how the excess pounds make you feel, emotionally and physically. Mention any weight-related health problems. Tell them that weight loss will be the most difficult thing you've ever tried and that you really need their support. List specific ways you'd like your family to help. For example, you might ask them to:

- Praise you when they see you eating foods on your plan.
- Organize social activities that do not focus on eating.
- Prepare foods that fit into the plan.
- Allow you time to prepare for the upcoming week.

Ask them not to:

- Eat your trigger foods in front of you.
- Purchase foods not included on the plan, especially ones you find tempting.
- Knowingly offer you foods that are not on the plan.
- Make negative comments about your weight, your past attempts at weight loss, or your level of willpower or motivation.

Plan, plan, and plan some more. Once you have a full mental handle on the eating plan, think about your upcoming week at work and at home. How and when do you usually eat? Which foods are around at work? Do you regularly see donuts and candy jars? Do you usually walk past a vending machine? Will you make your lunch or will you purchase it at work? If you will be packing a lunch for the first time, will you get up earlier in the morning to enable that to happen?

Take a look at your engagement calendar for work and personal appointments. Plan how you will prepare and purchase your meals for the coming week. Think of strategies that will help you handle tempting situations, such as business dinners or nights out with friends, and whether your strategy will be to eat a protein-rich snack ahead of time, decide on your dish without opening the menu, or ask the waiter not to bring the bread basket to the table.

Similarly, how will you stick with your eating habits on the days when life inevitably throws you a curve ball? What will you do if your child gets sick? (Consider having bagged greens ready to throw together with some protein for a quick meal.) What will you do if you're so busy that you don't get to the grocery store? (Maybe you'll choose to stock-pile five frozen meals for those moments when you just can't handle another errand.)

To succeed at weight loss, you can't let anything get in your way. You can't let anything stop you.

Make sure you are truly ready. Take the "Are You Ready?" quiz on page 88. If you are going through a divorce, buying a house, or changing careers, this may not be the best time in your life to try to lose weight. Think of it this way: if you were about to have a baby, would you choose that time to go back to school? If you were starting a new job, would you take on new volunteer work responsibilities?

Take life one challenge at a time. If your life is overly stressful right now, it's better to put off weight loss for a few months until you are ready to devote more attention to it. If you don't have the time or energy to commit to weight loss, it will become one more failure that will make you feel less confident the next time you try to lose weight. So finish any other big life projects first, even if they take 6 months or longer. Lose weight when you can devote time and energy to the project.

Get ready to work hard. Do you think that this will be difficult? It will. There's no getting around that. Sticking to a new way of eating may be the hardest thing you've ever done. Look at this as you would any big accomplishment, such as finishing your degree or seeing your first child head off to kindergarten (or college!). You know it will be hard, but you also know the payoff will be huge. With weight loss,

ARE YOU READY?

Answer each of the following questions with a yes or no to determine whether this is the best time for you to try to lose weight.

1. Are you devoting a lot of mental and physical energy to one or more huge life projects (a wedding, divorce, career change, geographic move, purchase of a new house, starting or expanding a family)?

    ☐ YES   ☐ NO

2. Are you willing to forgo certain types of foods and beverages when you're eating out, at a party, or doing something social with friends and family?

    ☐ YES   ☐ NO

3. Are you willing to temporarily curtail your social life if you find you lose control of your eating in social situations?

    ☐ YES   ☐ NO

4. Are you willing to change your behavior forever to lose weight and keep it off?

    ☐ YES   ☐ NO

5. Are you willing to make weight loss your top priority for the next few months or year (or however long it takes to reach your goal)?

    ☐ YES   ☐ NO

If you are ready to lose weight, you will have answered "no" to question #1. It's hard to lose weight if you are also tackling another big life change. You will have answered "yes" to the remaining questions. Many of these questions deal with social eating triggers. It's easy, when you're out with friends, to cheat and have a beer or two. Suddenly the beers lead to a few pretzels and the pretzels lead to potato skins, and off you go on a carb binge. You must be willing to stay focused and keep your goal of losing weight front and center. Weight loss must be the most important goal in your life for a very long time, and then, once you reach that goal, maintenance will take its place. Don't misunderstand us—you can still have fun. You just need to find nonfood-related ways to enjoy yourself. Maybe you can meet friends at a park or go to a cultural event together.

Finally, know that weight loss is a continuous life journey. You will probably never be able to return to your old way of eating. For the rest of your life, you will always be focused on eating the right balance of healthy carbs and fats in the form of wholesome foods.

If, based on your answers, you are not ready, put off weight loss for a few months, and then take the quiz again. When you are really ready to lose weight, you'll have crossed the great divide that separates wanting from doing. Once you are ready to change, you're ready to lose.

your payoff is a smaller body, better health, more energy, and improved self-confidence. It very well may be the most important challenge of your life, and when you get to that finish line you will be so glad you put in the effort.

Now, are *you* ready? Let's keep you alive. Let's get you healthy. Let's make you stronger, happier, and more energetic than ever. Turn to Chapter 6 to find out how.

THE REAL FOOD DIET

Our eating plans allow you to drop pounds and feel better by filling you up with lots of fiber, protein, and healthy fats, as well as daily indulgences. You will probably find that you must remind yourself to eat. That's how satisfied you'll feel between meals.

You'll choose from two levels of eating, Level 1 and Level 2. Choose the best plan for you based on your responses to the quizzes in Chapter 5. Each level provides you with a different level of carbohydrate consumption. Here's a brief description of each level.

LEVEL 1

This level provides you with up to 50 daily grams of carbohydrates. This amount of carbohydrates will help put your body in fat-burning mode, so the pounds will drop off quickly. Because the carbohydrate allotment is lower than in Level 2, you won't see as many carbohydrate indulgences. You'll choose from among chocolate, the recommended brands of bread, and low-glycemic fruit. Make sure you take note of your specific chocolate allowance. You'll also choose from avocado, nuts, or olives. Each day, you may indulge in a ricotta dessert. Sprinkle cinnamon, sugar-free chocolate syrup, nuts, or fruit (if this is your chosen indulgence) on top and enjoy!

LEVEL 2

Here you'll roughly triple your amount of carbohydrates, and with the increased carbs comes even more choices. You'll have the option of additional types of breads, oatmeal, *and* more indulgences like wine and chips. Similarly, you can continually eat olives *and* avocado *and* nuts.

REAL FOOD GUIDELINES

No matter which level you follow, we've done the number crunching for you by recommending minimum and maximum numbers of servings to eat of different types of foods. If you follow these recommendations, you'll automatically consume the right number of carbohydrate grams for your metabolism, without counting every single carbohydrate gram in the process. We have, however, provided you with the carbohydrate counts for suggested foods, as well as the carbohydrate range for each level. We hope this allows you to eventually gain an intuitive understanding of low-carb eating so you can customize the plan to your personal eating style over time.

Follow this advice:

Eat regularly. Never skip a meal. Going too long without eating can cause your blood sugar to drop too low, triggering cravings and overeating later on. If you have an insulin disadvantage or a thyroid disadvantage, this is especially important. Plan on eating six small meals a day to keep your blood sugar balanced. Always have convenient snacks on hand, such as hard-boiled eggs, precooked meatballs, cheese sticks, celery sticks, or turkey rolled with cheese. Eat early, and eat often. Doctor's orders.

Limit caffeine. We recommend you cut back on caffeinated beverages, especially coffee, for these reasons.

- Coffee is acidic and tends to promote yeast overgrowth.
- Caffeine triggers your stress response, raising cortisol and consequently insulin levels. This stress hormone jump also increases blood pressure.
- For many people, coffee disturbs sleep, and you need plenty of rest. This is especially true if you have an adrenal disadvantage.
- Research shows that caffeine produces alertness by reducing levels of a molecule called adenosine. Adenosine tends to promote better sleep and reduce the inflammation that can lead to heart disease, diabetes, and organ damage.
- Coffee and other caffeinated beverages may also harden your

arteries, increasing your risk of heart attack and stroke. When researchers gave 10 volunteers 100 milligrams of caffeine (the amount in one cup of coffee), wave reflection—a measure of artery stiffness—increased for at least 2 hours.

We recommend you reduce your consumption of caffeine as much as possible. Cut back on coffee, soda, and other caffeinated beverages. Drink no more than 1 cup (that's a measuring cup, and not a grande mug) of coffee a day, split between caffeinated and decaffeinated. If you get rebound headaches when you cut back on caffeine, take Tylenol (no more than 2 grams a day and if not contraindicated because of other medical problems or medicines you are taking) until the headaches subside.

Read labels carefully. Before buying any packaged food, take a look at the label. Specifically, look for the following.

1. **The list of ingredients.** Remember: We want you to eat clean. We recommend you do not purchase the food if you see the following terms on the list: *corn, soy, artificial colors, artificial sweetener,* or *partially hydrogenated*. Products are allowed to claim "trans free" on their packaging even when they contain up to 0.49 gram of trans fats. If an ingredients list has the words *partially hydrogenated*, the food contains trans fats. Another newer, just-as-bad fat is called interesterified oil. Manufacturers are using it in place of trans fats in processed foods, but it may raise blood sugar by 20 percent.

2. **The amount of carbohydrate versus the amount of fiber.** Calculate the product's fiber ratio by dividing the grams of fiber by the grams of carbohydrate. When comparing like foods—such as two different brands of crackers—choose the brand with the higher fiber score. If both brands score the same, choose the one with the fewest carbohydrate grams per serving.

3. **The amount of carbohydrate compared to the amount of fat and protein.** In an ideal world, your food would have a 1 to 1 ratio of each of these ingredients (for instance, 10 grams of carbohydrate, 10 grams of fat, and 10 grams of protein). Most foods, of course, contain more of one ingredient or another, but be wary

of foods that are close to 100 percent carbohydrates (for instance, 40 grams of carbohydrates, 2 grams of fat, and 2 grams of protein). Without enough protein and fat to slow digestion, these foods can wreak havoc on blood sugar and insulin levels, prompting hunger.

RECOMMENDED BRANDS

The following brands are as free as possible from harmful additives. In a few circumstances, no brand currently exists in a given food category that is completely free of additives. Syrups are a good example. In those cases, we've listed the cleanest brands available.

Crackers

Bran-a-crisp

Doctor Kracker pumpkin cheddar snack chips

GG Bran Scandinavian Crisp Bread

Kavli, 5 grain crispbread and crispy thin

RYVITA

Wasa Fiber Rye Crisp Bread

Tuna *(free of soy and lowest in mercury)*

365 Whole Foods Market Tongol tuna

Dairy and Yogurt *(no added sugar or high-fructose corn syrup)*

Blue Diamond Almond Breeze almond milk, unsweetened

Chobani Original Greek yogurt

FAGE Total Classic Greek yogurt, nonflavored

Pacific Organic Almond Milk, unsweetened (Level 2)

Stonyfield Farm Oikos Greek plain yogurt

Chocolate *(free of soy additives and lowest amounts of added sugar)*

DaVinci sugar-free syrup

Endangered Species

Green & Black's

Lindt chocolate (70% cocoa or higher)

Torani sugar free syrup

Vivani (72% cocoa or higher)

Nuts and Seeds *(high in fiber, low in added sugars)*

Blue Diamond

Bob's Red Mill Organic Golden Flaxseeds

David Original Sunflower Seeds

Kirkland

Nature's Path Ground Flaxseed

Let's Do Organic Unsweetened Coconut Lite

Planters

Pumpkorn Original and Adobo Chili

Shiloh Farms organic coconut

4. **The servings per container.** If you consume more than one serving, you're consuming more carbs than what is listed on the package.

To gain a better idea of how to make better choices based on the information on food labels, let's take a look at two brands of chocolate

Meat (no nitrates, harmful preservatives, or antibiotics)
Applegate Farms
Boar's Head golden roasted turkey
Coleman Natural
D'Artagnan wild game
Great Range bison
Laura's lean beef
Nature's Promise organic deli meat
Shelton's uncured chicken, beef, turkey franks, turkey sticks pepperoni, beef jerky, turkey bologna, turkey Italian sausage

Bread (free of high-fructose corn syrup and soy additives)
Alvarado Street Bakery Flax Bread
Ezekiel 4:9 bread
The Baker Whole Grain Flax Bread

Sauces, Spreads, and Spices
(no trans fats, no high-fructose corn syrup, and minimal added sugar)
Classico sauces (contain soy)
Cortland Valley organic sauerkraut
Del Monte diced tomatoes with mild green chilies
Gold's horseradish
Grace Jamaican curry powder
Grey Poupon Dijon
Marco Polo Caponata

Muir Glen tomato sauce
Tai Ethnic Gourmet Punjab Saag
Thai Kitchen Lite Coconut Milk
Trader Giotto's caponata

Dressings and Marinades
Annie's Naturals: Caesar dressing, Shiitake and Sesame Vinaigrette
Hidden Valley Ranch dressing (not all varieties; check labels)
Nature's Promise Teriyaki and Mandarin Orange Marinade (use 1 tablespoon per serving)
Newman's Own Olive Oil and Vinegar dressing
Trader Joe's Blue Cheese dressing

Beverages
Celestial Seasonings tea
Green & Black's organic hot chocolate drink (use ½ serving size)
Greens+, Original and Wild Berry Burst tea
Hint Premium Essence flavored water
MetroMint flavored water
Lipton tea
Numi tea
V8 100% vegetable juice

bars. What's the first ingredient listed for bar #1? Sugar. What about bar #2? Chocolate. Not only that, but bar #1 also contains a whole slew of non-chocolate-sounding ingredients, including soy and artificial flavors. Bar #2? It's chocolate.

Now, bar #1 certainly contains fewer calories and fat, and that's why most people would mistakenly choose it, but let's look at the carbs and fiber. Bar #1 has more carbs, 11 grams, whereas bar #2 has only 8 grams of carbs and three times more fiber. Bar #1's fiber ratio is a mere 9 percent, whereas #2 boasts a 37 percent fiber ratio. Finally, bar #2 contains a more balanced range of nutrients, with protein and fat to offset the carbs. Bar #1? Its carbohydrates are almost all sugar!

BRAND 1

Nutrition Facts

Serving Size 1 bar (17g)
Servings Per Container 7

Amount Per Serving

Calories 100   Calories from Fat 50

% Daily Value*

Total Fat 5g	8%
Saturated Fat 3g	20%
Trans Fat 0g	
Cholesterol 0mg	0%
Sodium 20mg	1%
Total Carbohydrate 11g	TK%
Dietary Fiber 1g	TK%
Sugars 9g	
Protein <1g	TK%

INGREDIENTS: sugar, chocolate, cocoa butter, cocoa processed with alkali, lactose, milk, soy lethicin, vanillin, artificial flavor

BRAND 2

Nutrition Facts

Serving Size 4 squares (40g)
Servings Per Container TK

Amount Per Serving

Calories 210   Calories from Fat 160

% Daily Value*

Total Fat 18g	28%
Saturated Fat 11g	55%
Trans Fat 0g	
Cholesterol 0mg	0%
Sodium 20mg	1%
Total Carbohydrate 8g	3%
Dietary Fiber 3g	12%
Sugars 5g	
Protein 4g	8%

INGREDIENTS: Chocolate, cocoa powder, cocoa butter, sugar, vanilla

Drink plenty of water. As you burn through your stores of carbohydrates, your body will release water in your urine. Make sure you drink plenty of water—80 to 100 ounces a day—and take a multivitamin to replace minerals that are sometimes lost during this diuretic stage of the diet. (See Chapter 9 for information about which multivitamin to take.)

Talk to your doctor before starting this eating approach. Ask your doctor to closely monitor your blood pressure, blood sugar, and insulin levels, *especially* if you are taking medication to control these health problems. Once your eating change starts to prompt results, you may need to reduce the dosage of the medications you take or stop taking some medicines altogether. If you are taking a diuretic, make sure your doctor knows that you will be embarking on an eating plan that has a temporary diuretic effect.

Don't take constipation lightly. It generally means you are not following the diet correctly and not consuming the recommended amounts of vegetables and water. If the constipation persists after you've upped your water and veggie intake, consider taking 500 to 1,000 milligrams of magnesium daily (as long as your kidney function is normal) to get things moving. (Do not do this if you have kidney disease.)

Breathe confidently. This eating level can sometimes result in bad breath as the body produces and burns ketones, by-products of fat metabolism. Your body creates these substances as it breaks down dietary and body fat. It recycles some of them, burning them for energy, too. And it also releases some through your urine, sweat, and breath. Unfortunately, they can be a bit smelly. Use breath-freshening products such as Breath Assure, drink lots of water, and chew on sprigs of parsley.

Avoid these foods if you have a yeast disadvantage. Whether you are in Level 1 or Level 2, refrain from eating any food that is fermented, pickled, or moldy, such as soy sauce, alcohol, vinegar, mushrooms, sour cream, sauerkraut, certain nuts (cashews, peanuts, pistachios), pickles, breads that contain yeast, and cheese. The exceptions are mozzarella and cream cheese; they are okay to eat.

Eat mindfully. Mindless eating can undo even the most diligent dieter's efforts. Make strides to remain aware of every bite that goes into your mouth—you'll not only enjoy your food more, but you'll also feel satisfied faster. To eat more mindfully, follow this advice:

- Eat meals while seated at a table. Do not eat while working, standing, or while preparing food in the kitchen.
- If you have children, make sure you notice any food you eat that they did not. It's all too easy to finish off the last bites of food from our kids' plates and then wonder why we aren't losing weight.

- Do not multitask while you eat. Turn off the TV. Put aside your book or magazine, and step away from the computer.
- Before you start eating, rate your hunger on a scale of 1 to 10. Take a few deep, relaxing breaths before inserting your first forkful into your mouth. Then, try to be completely aware of the taste and texture of the first forkful and periodic forkfuls throughout the meal. Savor your food. Chew it into a fine mush.
- About halfway through the meal, rate your hunger again. Once your hunger goes below 4 on your scale, stop eating. It takes a while for the hunger signals from your stomach to turn off. Within 20 minutes after finishing a meal, you'll probably drop from 4 to 0. If not, then go ahead and eat a little more until you feel satisfied.
- Be very aware of the taste and texture of your last forkful. The last one is critically important because it puts closure on your meal, preventing you from reaching for emotionally fueled seconds.
- Rate your hunger at the meal's end. This will help you to get in touch with your hunger and fullness signals, and it will keep you aware of the eating process. It also will heighten your enjoyment of eating.

Choose carbs with fiber. We allow bread, fruit, and other carbohydrate foods on all of our plans, but we recommend choosing higher fiber, naturally lower carb versions of these foods so you can maximize the nutritional value from the carbs you eat. To do so, calculate a food's fiber score. What's that? The fiber score is the number you get when you divide the grams of fiber in a food by the grams of carbohydrates and multiply by 100. (See a full list of foods with their fiber scores beginning on the opposite page.) Try to choose the foods with the highest scores in each food category, opting for the highest fiber veggies, fruits, grains, and other foods. (Keep in mind that you should combine high-carbohydrate foods with some protein and fat to minimize the blood sugar response.)

Put the focus on breakfast. This is the most important meal of the day to do right. If you start the day with a high-fiber, low-carbohydrate breakfast that contains protein, you will keep your blood sugar stable throughout the day. This, in turn, helps you make better choices all day.

FIBER SCORES

The fiber score is the number you get when you divide the grams of fiber in a food by the grams of carbohydrates and multiply by 100. Choose foods with the highest fiber scores within each category. For example, you'll see that most whole grain products have higher scores than refined grains and that minestrone soup is better than vegetable. Real foods that have lower fiber scores, such as blueberries, should not be avoided because they have antioxidants, vitamins, minerals, and other nutrients that make them an important part of a balanced diet.

FOOD	PORTION	CARBS (GRAMS)	FIBER (GRAMS)	FIBER RATIO	NOTE
Vegetables					
Romaine lettuce	1 cup	1.5	1	67	
Spinach, raw	1 cup	1.1	0.7	64	
Eggplant, raw	1 cup	5	3	60	
Mushroom, straw canned	½ cup	4.2	2.3	55	
Bibb lettuce	1 cup	1.2	0.6	50	
Boston lettuce	1 cup	1.2	0.6	50	
Iceberg lettuce	1 cup	2	1	50	
Greens+ drink	1 serving (3 tsp)	4	2	50	
Brussels sprouts, frozen	½ cup	6.5	3.2	49	
Cauliflower, raw	1 cup	4.3	2	47	
Celery, raw	1 cup	3.5	1.6	46	
Green beans, frozen	½ cup	4.5	2	44	
Broccoli, raw	1 cup	6.0	2.4	40	
Asparagus, canned, no salt added	½ cup	3.0	1.2	40	
Tomato, plum	1	2.4	0.8	33	
Cucumber	1 cup	2.9	0.9	31	

(continued)

FIBER SCORES (cont.)

FOOD	PORTION	CARBS (GRAMS)	FIBER (GRAMS)	FIBER RATIO	NOTE
Starchy Vegetables					
Peas, canned, no salt added, solids and liquids	½ cup	12.1	4.1	34	
Carrots	1¼ cups canned, no salt added, or 1 cup raw	6.6 12.3	2.2 3.6	33 29	
Sweet potato, baked	1 small	12.4	2	16	
Yam	½ cup cubed	21.4	3	14	
Corn, sweet, yellow, canned, no salt added	½ cup	15.4	1.6	10	
Potato, baked	1 small	29.2	3	10	
Potato, mashed	½ cup prepared from flakes without milk, whole milk and butter added	11.5	0.9	8	
Fruit					
Avocado, California	½	5.9	4.6	78	
Blackberries	½ cup	7.4	4.3	58	
Raspberries	½ cup	7.4	4	54	
Star fruit	1 medium	4.2	1.9	45	
Guava****	1 medium	7.9	3	38	
Asian pear	1 medium	13	4.4	34	
Olives	9 small	1.8	0.9	30	
Passion fruit	1 medium	10	3	30	
Strawberries	½ cup	5.9	1.5	25	
Pear	1 medium	27.5	5.5	20	
Orange	1 medium	15.4	3.1	20	
Papaya	½ cup	6.9	1.3	19	
Apricot	1	3.9	0.7	18	
Blueberries	½ cup	10.7	1.8	17	high in antioxidants

FOOD	PORTION	CARBS (GRAMS)	FIBER (GRAMS)	FIBER RATIO	NOTE
Apple	1 small	20.6	3.6	17	
Grapefruit	½ medium	13.1	2.0	15	
Casaba melon	½ cup	5.6	0.8	14	
Banana	1 medium	27	3.1	11	
Cantaloupe	1 cup diced	13.7	1.4	10	
Peach	1 small	12.9	1.2	9	
Watermelon	1 cup	11.6	0.6	5	
Grapes	1 cup	15.8	0.8	5	
Frozen Dinners					
Chicken Tandoori with spinach	1	8	4	50	670 mg sodium
Chicken Marsala with broccoli	1	10	2	20	530 mg sodium
Three cheese chicken	1	7.2	0.9	13	560 mg sodium
Oven-roasted chicken	1	37	2	5	770 mg sodium
Chicken portobello	1	48	2	4	560 mg sodium
Bread					
Damascus flaxseed roll-up	1	15	9	60	
The Baker whole grain flax	1 slice	8	3	38	
Food for Life The Original Bran for Life bread	1 slice	17	5	29	
Wonder Lite Wheat	2 slices	18	5	28	Contains corn syrup/ trans fats
Ezekiel 4:9 sprouted 100 percent whole grain bread	1 slice	15	3	20	
Arnold's 100 Calorie white bread	2 slices	21	4	19	Contains corn syrup/ trans fats

(continued)

FIBER SCORES *(cont.)*

FOOD	PORTION	CARBS (GRAMS)	FIBER (GRAMS)	FIBER RATIO	NOTE
Alvarado Street flax	2 slices	15	3	20	
Rye bread	1 slice	15.5	1.9	12	Contains corn syrup/ trans fats
Wonder white	1 slice	12	0.5	4	Contains corn syrup/ trans fats
Crackers					
Doctor Kracker pumpkin cheddar snack chips	8 chips	12	4	33	
Wasa fiber rye	1	8	2	25	
Ryvita dark rye	1	8	2	25	
Kavli thick cracker	1	7.5	1.5	20	
Kashi TLC party crackers Stone-grounds 7 grain	4	17	3	18	
Kavli thin cracker	1	4.3	0.7	16	
Triscuit	7	21	3	14	
Mary's Gone Crackers wheat free original	6	10.5	1.5	14	
Crispini Mediter-ranean Sesame snacking crisps	6 crisps	20	1	5	
Breakfast Cereals—Hot and Cold					
Quaker instant oats, high fiber maple and brown sugar	1 packet	34	10	29	
Roman Meal cream of rye	⅓ cup	25	5	20	
Wheatena	⅓ cup	35.7	6	17	
Bob's Red Mill steel cut oats	¼ cup	27	4	15	
Kellogg's Raisin Bran	1 cup	45	7	15	Contains high-fructose corn syrup

FOOD	PORTION	CARBS (GRAMS)	FIBER (GRAMS)	FIBER RATIO	NOTE
Quaker 1 minute oats	½ cup dry	27	4	14	
Tesco Scottish porridge oats	½ cup	30	4	13	
Multigrain Cheerios	1 cup	23	3	13	
US Mills Farina	1 cup	22	1	4	
Pasta					
Ronzoni Smart Taste spaghetti	2 oz	43	6.3	15	
Ronzoni Healthy Harvest whole wheat pasta	2 oz	42	6	14	
Eden organic spelt ribbons	½ cup	41	5	12	
Dreamfields rotini	2 oz	42	5	12	
Barilla Plus spaghetti	2 oz	38	4	10	
Ancient Harvest quinoa spaghetti	2 oz	35	2.5	7	
Bionaturae organic 100% whole wheat gobbetti	2 oz	42	3	7	
Pasta Joy Ready spinach style brown rice pasta	2 oz	44	2	4	
Rice and Grains					
Kashi 7 whole grain pilaf	½ cup	30	6	20	
Quinoa	½ cup cooked	19.7	2.6	13	
Wild rice	½ cup cooked	17.5	1.5	9	
Brown rice	½ cup cooked	22.4	1.8	8	
Instant brown rice	½ cup cooked	33	2	6	
Couscous	½ cup cooked	18.3	1.1	6	

(continued)

FIBER SCORES (cont.)

FOOD	PORTION	CARBS (GRAMS)	FIBER (GRAMS)	FIBER RATIO	NOTE
Chocolate					
Vivani 85% cacao	2.5 oz .	5.9	5.3	90	
Vivani 70% cacao	2.5 oz	11	4.5	41	
Lindt 85% cocoa dark chocolate	4 squares	8	3	37	
Rapunzel bittersweet	½ bar	12	4	33	
Dagoba Mon Cheri 72% cacao	½ bar	14	4	28	
Hershey's 65% cacao	1.4 oz	18	4	28	
Ghirardelli Twilight Delight 72% cacao	3 pieces	17	4	23	
Lindt 70% cocoa	3 squares	10	2	20	
Chocolove 65% cocoa	⅓ bar	15	3	20	
Vosges Creole bar	3 squares	16	3	18	
Hershey's 100 calorie dark chocolate bar	1 bar	11	1	9	
Newman's Own sweet dark espresso	⅓ bar	14	1	7	
Nuts and Nut Butters					
Pecans	19 halves	4	2.7	68	
Almonds	1 oz	5.4	3.3	61	
Macadamias	1 oz	4.0	2.4	60	
Coconut	1 oz	4.3	2.5	58	
Hazelnuts	1 oz	4.7	2.7	57	
Almond butter	2 tbsp	6	3	50	
Walnuts	1 oz	3.8	1.9	50	
Peanut butter, chunky	2 tbsp	6.9	2.6	38	
Dry-roasted peanuts	1 oz	6.0	2.2	37	
Peanut butter, smooth	2 tbsp	6.4	1.9	30	

FOOD	PORTION	CARBS (GRAMS)	FIBER (GRAMS)	FIBER RATIO	NOTE
Pine nuts	1 oz	3.7	1	27	
Peanut butter, reduced fat	2 tbsp	10	1.5	10	
Cashews	1 oz	9.2	0.9	10	
Cashew butter	2 tbsp	8.8	0.6	7	
Beans and Legumes					
Lentil	¼ cup	28.8	14.7	50	
Kidney, canned	½ cup	20.5	6.8	33	
Refried	½ cup	19.5	6.7	33	
Lima	½ cup	18	5.8	32	
Pinto	½ cup	18.3	5.5	30	
Soy	½ cup	28.5	8.7	30	
Chickpea	¼ cup	30	8.7	29	
Great Northern	½ cup	19	5	26	
Black	¼ cup	30	7.4	25	
Baked	¼ cup	30	7.5	25	
Navy	½ cup	26.8	6.7	24	
Pancakes					
Pancakes prepared from Arrowhead Mills oat bran pancake and waffle mix	2 (5-inch) cakes	27	3	11	
Pancakes prepared from mix, refined grain	1 medium cake	15	1	6	
Dips, Toppings, and Dressings					
Genji all natural ginger miso dressing	2 tbsp	2	0	0	
Cara Mia marinated mushrooms with garlic	4 pieces	1	0	0	
Hannah bruschetta	½ cup	6	0	0	contains additives

(continued)

FIBER SCORES (cont.)

FOOD	PORTION	CARBS (GRAMS)	FIBER (GRAMS)	FIBER RATIO	NOTE
Hannah tzatziki	1 tbsp	1	0	0	Contains additives
Hannah spinach dip	2 tbsp	3	0	0	
Misc. Prepared Foods					
Muir Glen minestrone soup	½ can	19	5	26	
V8 100% vegetable juice	1 can	10	2	20	
Campbell's Healthy Request tomato juice	1 can	10	2	20	
Muir Glen garden vegetable soup	½ can	16	3	19	
Nasoya Tofu	1 cup	2.3	0.4	17	
Thai Kitchen organic lite coconut milk	2 oz	1	0	0	

Include vegetables at every meal. Vegetables contain fiber, so they fill you up and keep you regular. Vegetables also contain important antioxidants, nutrients that protect your cells from oxidative damage. For each level of the diet, you'll find a number of recipes that creatively sneak fiber-rich vegetables into everyday foods such as grilled cheese and even hamburgers. Add more veggies by rounding out lunch and dinner with side salads and heaping servings of steamed or sautéed broccoli, cauliflower, greens, or another veggie of your choice.

Never give up. If you go beyond your daily recommended indulgence and have dessert or a couple of glasses of wine one night, *you have not blown it*! Use the splurge as motivation to get yourself back on track. Rather than using it as an excuse to have a donut for breakfast ("*I cheated last night, I might as well keep cheating*"), simply tell yourself that you will recommit, and make up for it by following the Level 1 approach flawlessly the next day, even if you are supposed to follow Level 2.

7

LEVEL 1

Limiting carbohydrates will trigger your body to burn through its stores of glycogen and carbohydrate. Once your body depletes these reserves—a process that takes roughly 2 to 3 days, depending on your activity level—your body will preferentially burn fat for fuel, and your weight will drop quickly. This switch to fat burning will help reduce insulin levels, quieting your hunger and allowing you to feel more satisfied.

Level 1 is healthy. It provides you with plenty of fiber and nutrition from vegetables. You can follow it for weeks, months, and even years—and some of our clients have done just that. You do not *have* to transition to Level 2 eating.

The length of time you choose to follow Level 1 will depend on your body and your level of motivation. Here's what we recommend:

- **In general, follow the Level 1 plan for at least 2 weeks.**
- **If you have an insulin disadvantage,** follow Level 1 as closely as possible and stick with it for at least a month before modifying the plan or progressing to Level 2.
- **If you feel deprived and ready to quit the plan altogether,** move up to Level 2 as needed. It's okay, from time to time, to jump up to Level 2. If you will be on vacation or celebrating the holidays, or you just need more flexibility, don't torture yourself—just don't overdo it. Plan your indulgences, but stay as close as possible to the rest of the plan. You will probably lose weight more slowly or perhaps not at all. Your weight loss should resume at its previous rate

once you start back on Level 1 again. If you are on vacation, try going back to Level 1 on your last day to prepare yourself for getting home and back on the plan. Maintaining control and getting with the program as soon as possible is critical. This gets you used to making choices and practicing control. Allow yourself some slack, recognize this, and then pull back again when you're ready to buckle down.

There's no reason to put yourself through hell to lose weight. This is *your* plan!

WHAT TO EAT ON LEVEL 1

You'll find minimum and maximum serving sizes for specific types of foods. Eating less than the minimum daily amounts of the required foods can be a recipe for frustration, hunger, cravings, and disaster. The protein offers a wealth of important nutrients for total-body health; the vegetables provide not only nutrients and antioxidants, but also plenty of appetite-suppressing fiber. Both help keep you satisfied. Don't skimp. If you consistently find that you cannot meet the plan's vegetable quota, you may supplement your vegetable intake with a "green drink." Sold in health food stores and online, these drinks provide the nutritional benefits of many different vegetables. See our Vanilla Almond or Strawberry Sensation Smoothies (pages 228 and 229), in which a green drink is one of the ingredients. Ideally, we'd like you to eat real food. Realistically, we know that these drinks help fill in the gaps for most people.

Here's some other important advice to help you get the full benefits and optimal results from the Level 1 diet.

Stick with the recommended portions of added fats. Don't worry about how much fat you consume from whole foods such as meat, fatty fruits and vegetables (such as avocados), and eggs. When you consume a diet composed of whole foods, you will naturally consume the right balance of fats, proteins, and carbs. Added fats in the form of olive oil, butter, and ghee, however, can easily overload your diet with fat and calories. Our daily allotment of these added fats is quite generous. Use oils only as dressings for salads and to lightly coat a pan when cooking. Do not use fats for deep-fat frying.

OLIVE OIL: THE WHOLE STORY

Unlike other types of vegetable oils, the extra virgin variety of olive oil does not undergo high-temperature processing that can create free radicals, dangerous chemicals that can attack cells and damage tissue. Instead, it is made by crushing olives between stone or steel. This preserves the beneficial fatty acids and natural preservatives in the oil. Olive oil needs to be packaged in an opaque (not clear) container to retain the freshness of its antioxidants, though. Look for the unfiltered type. Once you pour it from the bottle, watch to make sure the oil is dark. The lighter the color, the more the oil has been processed. Because heat can destroy its antioxidants and turn it rancid, we recommend you do not use olive oil in cooking. Use it only to drizzle over food *after* cooking, such as on roasted peppers or asparagus. For cooking, use coconut oil, ghee, butter, grapeseed oil, walnut oil, or high-heat cooking oil. For the same reasons that you shouldn't cook with it, do not keep olive oil for long periods of time. Rather than purchasing enormous bottles, buy the smallest bottle offered.

Watch your cheese portions. We recommend you eat only 3 to 4 ounces daily, for many reasons. Cheese is easy to overeat. Many people head to the fridge thinking that they will have just one slice, then find they can't stop until they've polished off a half pound. Dairy products contain carbohydrate in the form of lactose. Although cheese is lower in lactose than milk is (which is why we allow cheese at all), it's still not a food that you can eat without limits. Cheese also contains high amounts of salt, which can raise blood pressure and cause bloating in susceptible people. When you bloat from excess salt, you retain water. Your weight does not go down on the scale and you feel pudgy around the middle. If you have done a low-carb diet in the past and your LDL levels have not fallen, cheese may have been one of the culprits.

Measure your nuts. At one time, nuts were considered antithetical to weight loss, but recent research has confirmed that nuts are a tremendous ally in the fight against extra pounds—not to mention heart disease, diabetes, and cancer. Consider:

- Many nuts, such as pecans, sunflower seeds, and Brazil nuts, are rich in arginine, a precursor of nitric oxide, which causes blood vessel relaxation. Eating nuts can help keep your artery walls flexible and healthy and can lessen your chances of developing blood clots that lead to fatal heart attacks.

- One large study found that women who never or almost never ate nuts were significantly more likely to develop diabetes than were those who ate nuts more often—and the more nuts they ate, the further their risk declined.
- A study published in the journal *Circulation* found that adding 25 almonds a day reduced LDL cholesterol by 4 percent and raised HDL by 5 percent after just 1 month.
- Many nuts are packed with cancer-fighting antioxidants such as quercetin and kaempferol.
- Walnuts are one of the best vegetable sources of omega-3s, with 1 ounce of the nuts providing well over 1 gram of this essential fatty acid, as well as almost 2 grams of protein. Walnuts also have tryptophan, an amino acid that aids sleep.
- One study of vegetarians found those who ate nuts at least five times a week cut their risk of dying from heart disease in half versus those who rarely ate them; another review of large-scale studies determined that eating nuts five times a week can reduce your risk of heart disease by up to 39 percent.

Like cheese, however, nuts contain carbohydrate and are easy to over-eat. You start with a handful (the recommended 1-ounce serving size being roughly equal to the amount of nuts that will fit in your cupped hand) and you end up finishing off an entire jar or bag. So rather than eat them as a snack, we recommend you put them on top of salads or mix them into meals. Carefully measure them, using them as a topping or eating them one at a time if you do chose them as a snack. This can help prevent overeating.

Choose organic, nitrate-free meat whenever possible. If you cannot afford these options or they are not available, do the best you can.

Choose the types of fish listed on page 52. These are the varieties that are lowest in mercury and other contaminants.

Enliven meals with olives. Olives are such a nutritional power-house that we've added them to your daily food plan right from the start. They are great snack foods. Three-quarters of the caloric content from olives comes from healthful monounsaturated fat that can lower levels of bad LDL cholesterol and raise good HDL. In addition:

- Olives are a rich source of vitamin E, a fat-soluble antioxidant that disarms dangerous free radicals and helps prevent colon cancer.

COCONUT OIL CURES

You've probably heard that you should avoid coconut oil because it's high in saturated fat. Although it's true that the type of fat in coconut oil is mostly saturated, it's not true that you need to avoid it. Studies show that this type of oil has anti-inflammatory properties. It has been shown that the medium-chain triglycerides—the specific type of saturated fat in coconut oil—are more easily burned for energy than are other sources of fat. Studies done on animals show that coconut oil tends to reduce appetite and speed metabolism.

But won't it raise cholesterol? No. Again, the type of saturated fat in coconut oil has been shown to *reduce* the risk for heart disease, not raise it. Unlike olive oil, this oil is stable when heated, making it ideal to use in cooking. For these reasons, you'll see that we recommend coconut oil in many of the recipes in this book. (You may also use unsalted butter, ghee, or another high-heat cooking oil.)

- The polyphenols and flavonoids in olives fight inflammation in the body, which can relieve the symptoms of asthma and arthritis.
- Olives' good fat helps stabilize blood sugar and even helps reverse insulin resistance.
- Olives' monounsaturated fats can also help prevent arterial plaque from building up on artery walls, reducing the risk of heart disease.

Some people find that including olives in their daily eating routine cuts out their craving for other salty snacks. Stick to the 14 recommended olives, though, especially if you have high blood pressure, because of the high salt content—1 ounce of pitted, brine-cured olives packs 462 milligrams of sodium, one-fifth of your daily maximum for this nutrient.

Pucker up for lemon juice. Among numerous other health benefits, the acidic nature of lemon juice blunts blood sugar spikes and helps control the release of energy after a meal. Also:

- Lemon juice is an excellent source of vitamin C—a ¼ cup of lemon juice, just 15 calories' worth, packs almost 50 percent of your daily value.
- One study in the journal *Public Health Nutrition* found that low vitamin C increased the likelihood of developing abdominal fat by 131 percent.

■ Another study of more than 20,000 people showed that people who ate the most vitamin C–rich foods were three times less likely to develop arthritis than those who ate the least.

■ Vitamin C helps prevent cholesterol from sticking to cell walls, and lemon's flavonoids attack free radicals and protect against cancer.

Many of our patients use lemon juice to add zesty flavor to sautéed greens and salads. If you were a diet soda addict before starting the plan, add lemon juice to sparkling water or seltzer for a very refreshing and much healthier alternative.

Add seasonings. Experiment with low-carb, low-calorie seasonings such as pepper, garlic, onion powder, ginger, and many other herbs and spices.

Indulge daily. You'll see we include chocolate on this meal plan. Have it! This sweet treat will not blow your diet—and in fact, by satisfying your cravings, it may help you stay with the program. If you're in the mood for something a little different, layer yogurt and fruit in a glass to make a parfait. Our patients love this dessert.

Pair carbs with fat and protein. Always consume bread or fruit along with protein and fat. This will limit its effect on blood sugar and help fill you up. For example, have fruit with ricotta cheese or fresh whipped cream (not the canned variety), or spread peanut or almond butter on bread.

LEVEL 1 DAILY PLAN

EAT THESE DAILY	VARIETIES	SERVING SIZES/DAY	CARBOHYDRATES PER SERVING (GRAMS)
Protein foods	Beef Eggs Fish and shellfish (see page 52 for low-mercury varieties) Lamb Pork Poultry Nitrate-free sausages and franks Nitrate-free deli meat Tofu Wild game: venison, ostrich, bison	4 oz at breakfast (1 large egg = 2 oz) 4 to 8 oz at lunch and dinner (3 oz meat, poultry, or fish = size of a deck of cards) 2 oz for snacks	0 g per oz

EAT THESE DAILY	VARIETIES	SERVING SIZES/DAY	CARBOHYDRATES PER SERVING (GRAMS)
Leafy and green vegetables	Arugula Beet greens Bok choy Broccoli rabe Butterhead lettuce Celery Chard Collards Cucumber Endive Escarole Kale Mizuna Mustard greens Radicchio Red leaf lettuce Romaine Shallots Sorrel Spinach Turnip greens Watercress	3 to 5 cups raw (1 cup = 4 lettuce leaves)	1 g per cup
Vegetables	Artichoke Asparagus Bell peppers Broccoli Brussels sprouts Cabbage Cauliflower Chicory Eggplant Garlic Green beans Kohlrabi Leeks Onions Mushroom Pickles (1 large) Tomato Zucchini	1 cup raw vegetables OR 4 oz tomato or vegetable juice + ½ cup raw vegetables	7 to 15 g per cup

EAT THESE DAILY	VARIETIES	SERVING SIZES/DAY	CARBOHYDRATES PER SERVING (GRAMS)
Dairy foods	Almond milk, unsweetened (½ cup) Any sliced or stick cheese (1 stick or 1 slice) Cottage cheese (¼ cup) Cream (1 oz) Cream cheese (1 Tbsp) Greek yogurt (½ cup) Ricotta cheese (¼ cup)	3 to 4 oz	1 per ½ cup or 1 oz
Bread or fruit	**Recommended brands of bread and crackers** (see page 94)* **Fruit:** Apple Apricots (4 medium) Blackberries Blueberries (½ cup) Cantaloupe (⅛ large) Cherries (20 medium) Grapefruit (½) Orange Peach Pear Pineapple, fresh (½ cup diced) Plum Raspberries Strawberries Watermelon	2 slices bread or 2 crackers OR 1 small whole fruit or ¾ cup berries or diced fruit	15 g per oz
Snacks	Avocado (½ small) Nuts, all varieties Olives, all varieties (14)	1 oz nuts (1 oz = 23 whole almonds, 19 pecan halves, 1 Tbsp flaxseed, 1 Tbsp peanut or other nut butter)	5 g per Tbsp
Chocolate	Sugar-free chocolate syrup Dark chocolate, 85% cocoa + 4 to 6 nuts (part of the above serving)	1 Tbsp OR 2 squares	0 to 5 g per Tbsp

EAT THESE DAILY	VARIETIES	SERVING SIZES/DAY	CARBOHYDRATES PER SERVING (GRAMS)
Added fats	**For salad dressing:** Olive oil or recommended dressings (see page 95) **For cooking and spreads:** Butter unsalted Coconut oil Ghee Grapeseed oil High-heat cooking oil Mayonnaise Walnut oil	4 to 5½ Tbsp	0 g per Tbsp
Toppings and flavorings	Lemon or lime juice Coconut, unsweetened and additive-free Condiments, unsweetened and additive-free, such as mustard, horseradish, caponata, bruschetta (use serving size on label)	2 oz lemon or lime juice ½ cup coconut	1 to 5 g per oz

* For the Ezekiel 4:9 bread, please note that one 1-oz serving is 1 slice.

SAMPLE MEAL PLANS

Use the following 7 days' worth of menus as a guide. Feel free to mix and match various meals to create your own customized plans, or just use these as inspiration.

DAY 1

MORNING SNACK

4 large celery stalks with 2 tablespoons peanut butter or cream cheese

Michelle's Relaxing Mocktail (page 230)

BRUNCH

Spinach and Feta Omelet (page 228)

SNACK

4 ounces roast beef with horseradish

DINNER

Salad made with:

- 3 cups romaine lettuce
- 1 ounce chopped red pepper
- 1 ounce walnuts
- 1 tablespoon olive oil
- ½ tablespoon lemon juice
- 6 ounces roasted, chopped chicken
- ½ cup broccoli

SNACK

Tuna salad made with:

- 3 ounces tuna
- 2 tablespoons mayonnaise

Sharon's Chocolate Dream (page 230)

DAY 2

BREAKFAST

Vanilla Almond Smoothie (page 228)

SNACK

2 turkey franks with 1 ounce sauerkraut

LUNCH

Salad made with:
- 2 cups romaine
- 4 ounces sliced turkey
- ¼ avocado, sliced
- 2 tomato wedges
- 2 ounces blue cheese
- 1 tablespoon Caesar dressing

SNACK

2 roasted chicken drumsticks with 1 tablespoon
blue cheese dressing

DINNER
- 1 cup beef broth
- 6 ounces broiled T-bone steak
- 2 cups bok choy, ½ cup steamed Mashed Cauliflower
(page 233)

SNACK

3 stalks celery

Egg salad made with:
- 2 large hard-boiled eggs
- 1 tablespoon mayonnaise

Note: If your breakfast keeps you full until lunch, do not stuff yourself
by eating the turkey franks.

DAY 3

BREAKFAST

4 ounces smoked salmon

2 tablespoons cream cheese

2 ounces diced cucumber

SNACK

1 tablespoon almond butter

3 celery stalks

LUNCH

Salad made with:
- 1 cup lettuce
- ½ tablespoon olive oil
- 1 tablespoon lemon juice

4 ounces hamburger (85% lean ground round) topped with:
- 1 tablespoon mayonnaise
- 2 teaspoons mustard
- 1 tablespoon sautéed onion
- 1 ounce cooked portobello mushroom
- ½ avocado, sliced

SNACK

1 slice lite extra-firm tofu mixed with:
- 1 ounce garlic and onion tomato sauce
- 1 slice part–skim mozzarella, melted on top

DINNER

2 cups raw bok choy sautéed in 1 tablespoon coconut oil

Mexican Chicken Stir-Fry (page 240)

SNACK

½ cup whole strawberries

2 tablespoons heavy cream, whipped

DAY 4

BREAKFAST

Eggs Florentine (page 229)

SNACK

2 ounces Baked Cheese (page 235)

⅓ cup eggplant caponata

LUNCH

3 cups lettuce with 2 tablespoons Caesar dressing

2 turkey franks with 1 tablespoon mustard

SNACK

½ avocado, sliced

2 ounces boiled shrimp mixed with ½ tablespoon mustard

DINNER

Chicken vegetable soup made with:
- 2 cups chicken broth
- ½ cup frozen garden vegetable stir-fry

Curry Chicken (page 240)

¼ cup cooked green beans mixed with ¼ cup bruschetta

SNACK

2 slices turkey rolled with:
- 1 tablespoon mayonnaise
- 3 leaves red leaf lettuce

DAY 5

BREAKFAST

1 slice French Toast (page 227), ½ serving

2 turkey franks

SNACK

1 tablespoon almond butter with

3 celery stalks

LUNCH

6 ounces salmon kebobs made with:

- 20 strips green pepper
- ½ cup cubed eggplant
- 1 tablespoon coconut oil
- 1 teaspoon oregano
- 1 minced garlic clove for basting

Salad made with:

- 2 cups butterhead lettuce
- ¼ cup cherry tomatoes
- 1 tablespoon olive oil and vinegar dressing

SNACK

2 string cheese sticks

DINNER

6 ounces Steak Fajitas (page 236)

1½ cups spinach sautéed with:

- 1 teaspoon unsalted butter
- 1 cup beef broth

SNACK

8 ounces orange flavored seltzer

Chicken salad made with:

- 3 ounces cooked chicken
- 1 tablespoon mayonnaise

DAY 6

BREAKFAST

3 ounces cottage cheese

3 ounces pineapple

SNACK

3 ounces cooked chicken breast strips mixed with 2 tablespoons vinaigrette

LUNCH

French onion soup made with:

- 2 cups Pacific beef broth
- ¼ cup diced onion
- 1 ounce melted mozzarella cheese

Salad made with:

- 3 cups romaine lettuce
- 7 olives
- 1 tablespoon olive oil and vinegar dressing

5 ounces broiled T-bone steak

SNACK

2 hard-boiled eggs

DINNER

6 ounces cooked salmon encrusted with 1 tablespoon flaxseed

2 cups collard greens cooked with 1 tablespoon butter

½ cup cooked spaghetti squash mixed with 1 teaspoon butter

SNACK

Sharon's Chocolate Dream (page 230)

1 tablespoon almond butter

DAY 7

BREAKFAST

Turkey roll-up made with:
- 4 ounces turkey
- 1 ounce cheese
- 4 red leaf lettuce leaves

SNACK

3 ounces cottage cheese

½ ounce walnuts

LUNCH

4 ounces sole

Shrimp salad made with:
- 8 large grilled shrimp
- ¼ cup diced, peeled cucumber
- ½ cup boiled asparagus
- 2 cups spinach
- 4 tablespoons vinaigrette

SNACK

2 turkey franks

1 tablespoon mustard

DINNER

1 cup sliced cucumber dipped in 4 tablespoons Ranch dressing

6 ounce burger (85% lean ground beef)

½ cup cooked Brussels sprouts

SNACK

2 squares 85% cacao chocolate

½ ounce almonds

1 cup decaf hazelnut coffee with 1 ounce cream

RESTAURANT SUGGESTIONS

When eating out, always ask how your meal will be prepared. Grill your waiter or waitress about sauces, dressings, and fillers. Meatballs, for example, might be a great low-carbohydrate choice, but only if they are made without bread crumbs. A piece of fish might contain hidden carbs if the sauce on top of it is made with sugar. When looking at the menu, look for words such as scampi, garlic and oil, grilled, poached, braised, baked, or broiled. Also, remember to get more vegetables, either as a salad or as a side dish. Few restaurants serve enough with the meal.

The following dishes are usually low in carbohydrates:

Chinese: Choose steamed options whenever possible, adding low-sodium soy sauce at the table. Substitute steamed vegetables for the rice that would normally come with your meal. Beware of cornstarch, thickening agents, and sugar, as well as dishes that may contain peas or baby corn.

Beef with assorted sautéed vegetables

Beef with bamboo shoots

Lamb with scallions

Pepper steak with steamed mixed vegetables

Satay beef

Satay chicken

Spareribs (pat off the sauce)

Steamed mixed vegetables

Vegetable and bean curd soup (omit this choice if you have a yeast disadvantage)

Japanese: As with Chinese, avoid the rice that often comes with the meal and ask a lot of questions about sauces.

Hibachi chicken, shrimp, or beef with vegetables

Miso soup (don't eat this if you have a yeast disadvantage)

Sautéed or stir-fried vegetables

Sushi or sashimi without rice (substitute cucumbers for the rice)

Italian: Substitute a side salad or side of vegetables for the pasta that accompanies any main course. Ask the server not to bring bread.

If you do not eat Italian very often, you might splurge by allowing yourself a controlled amount of a cherished high-carb food, but choose it carefully and intentionally. Do you want a side dish of pasta, half a dessert, or a glass of wine? Choose only one splurge, not all three. Also, know that most commercial pasta sauces contain a great deal of sugar.

Appetizers

Caesar salad (without croutons)

Mussels marinara

Scungilli salad

Tomato with fresh mozzarella

Entrees

Calamari alla marinara (calamari in marinara sauce)

Eggplant, sausage, meatball, or chicken parmigiana (minus any fried bread crumbs)

Fish or chicken over sautéed spinach or broccoli rabe

Meatballs (no bread)

Sausage

Shrimp scampi with sautéed vegetables

Veal sautéed in garlic and oil

Zuppa di pesce (clams, mussels, scungilli, and shrimp in marinara sauce)

Deli: Avoid the bread that comes with sandwiches, wraps, and hoagies, eating only the insides or asking for the meat without the bread. Ask for a salad, even if it is not a menu option.

Eat the insides of any sandwich; omit the bread

Chef's salad

Meatballs

Sausage

Indian: Omit the rice that may come with your meal, and ask questions about how sauces are prepared. Look for sauces that do not contain yogurt or cornstarch and main courses that do not contain peas, potatoes, or legumes, all of which are common in Indian cooking.

Mashed eggplant (Baigan Ka Bharta)

Sheek kebab

Spinach curry with cheese

Tandoori chicken

Middle Eastern: Avoid falafel, baklava, bulgur wheat, and grape leaves. Good choices include the following:

Baba ghannouj

Grilled meat (chicken, beef, lamb)

Hummus

Shish kebab

Family style: Many family-style restaurants offer an assortment of meals that will work for Level 1. Substitute a side of vegetables or a salad for french fries, pasta, baked potato, and any other starch that may come with your meal. The menus at these restaurants vary. Below are some typical options.

Big salads, as long as you omit any nuts, croutons, fried tortilla crisps, peas, corn, or beans that may come with the salad

Chicken with steamed or sautéed vegetables

Double cheeseburger, stuffing the lettuce, tomato, and other toppings between the patties and using the patties as your "bun"

Hamburger without the bun (eat with a knife and fork or use two slices of tomato as a bun; ask for guacamole to liven it up)

Salmon with steamed or sautéed vegetables

Steak (substitute broccoli or another vegetable for the potato)

Fast food: Ask to see the list of ingredients for all fast food options before ordering. Many fast food meals contain hidden trans fats. For example, we were surprised to learn that the scrambled eggs at one popular fast food chain contained partially hydrogenated oils. Substitute a side salad for fries.

Angus hamburger (omit the bun and eat with a knife and fork or bring your own bread)

Grilled chicken (no bun)

Salad with oil and vinegar (Avoid vinegar if you have a yeast dis-advantage). Omit any nuts, croutons, fried tortilla crisps, corn, or beans that may come with the salad.

Scrambled eggs

Mexican: Ask the server to bring veggies to dip into salsa instead of the typical tortilla chips, or order a protein-rich appetizer such as shrimp. Substitute a vegetable side or a salad for the rice and beans that normally accompany a meal.

Fajitas (omit the tortilla wraps)

Mesquite grilled fish, steak, or chicken

Taco salad (omit the taco shell)

8

LEVEL 2

Welcome to Level 2. You will start with this level if you have a thyroid or an adrenal disadvantage or if you have a yeast disadvantage *and* are not overweight. You can also start at Level 2 if you are a carb-o-holic who is not ready for the strictness of Level 1 or if you have only 5 to 10 pounds to lose. Also, if you have yeast but are close to your ideal weight, start here. Rather than go cold turkey, start on this plan, and slowly remove carbs until you've adjusted to Level 1 eating.

Otherwise, you will start at Level 1, moving up to Level 2 after at least 2 weeks or until you've lost at least 20 percent of your starting weight.

Before you can decide whether you can use Level 2 successfully, you must determine what type of eater you are. Consider the following statements:

1. **I can eat small portions of bread, cookies, and other carbohydrate foods and stop.** I can go for weeks without eating sweets, starches (bread or crackers), or fruit and I don't miss them.

2. **Once I eat an indulgence food (ice cream, cookies, brownies, etc.),** I can't stop eating. One cookie becomes 10 cookies. One scoop of ice cream becomes the entire container. I need to follow a diet as directed—with not one cheat—or I might as well not follow it at all.

Which statement resonates more for you? If it's statement #1, you will probably be able to flawlessly transition to Level 2 eating. If statement #2 rings true, we recommend you transition to Level 2 with caution. Following Level 2 involves a certain degree of self-trust—you have to believe in your ability to hold yourself to the recommended serving sizes of the luxury foods. After all, this is not about *eating* perfectly; it's about *following the plan* consistently. The luxury foods are in there for a reason, so using them is not a slipup—you're simply following doctor's orders. Eating these foods in the amounts we recommend will *not* wreck your diet in any way. They are not forbidden foods. They are encouraged so you do not feel deprived! It's not realistic to try to forgo eating your favorite foods for the rest of your life. For your long-term success, you need to learn how to eat these foods with control and in moderation. If you continually lose control, however, you may be the type of person who does better with zero indulgence. If that's the case, go back to Level 1 until you feel you have more control. Level 1 is a healthy and balanced eating plan. You can stay on it for the rest of your life if need be.

Second, it may help to make a list of all of the foods you consider to be "trigger foods." These are the foods that cause you to lose control. When you see them sitting on a table, you feel fear. When you eat them, you barely enjoy the experience because you're filled with guilt. Make a list of those foods now, and then look over the Level 2 plans. Are those foods included on these plans? If so, put off incorporating those foods into your daily repertoire for a while, until you feel more in control. You should not look to any food as an emotional crutch. If you see food as sustenance, you will be able to forgo eating any food for a given amount of time and then bring it back, without losing control.

Try an experiment in a controlled setting to see how much control you really do have. Say your trigger food is ice cream. Go with a friend to an ice cream store. Order a kid's size scoop in a cup. Walk outside the store (to remove the temptation of getting another scoop). Eat the ice cream slowly. Enjoy every bite. It's your friend's job to make sure you do not walk back up to the counter and order another scoop. See how you do. If you do not feel the least bit tempted to order another scoop, you've successfully transitioned your mind-set to Level 2 eating. Know that this is an accomplishment and stay on the plan the rest of the day. On the other hand, if your friend has to drag you out of the store as you yell a string of curse words, wait a few more months before trying the experiment again—and you should probably stay away from indulging in ice cream.

Keep a journal about each experiment you try. We know, we know. It's time-consuming and inconvenient. Can you try to do it for the first month, until you break the bad habit of guilt-filled eating? Carry a small notebook with you and whenever you indulge in a luxury food, write it down. Jot down how much you ate and how you felt as you ate. Rate your sense of control on a scale of 1 to 10. Periodically look over the entries in your diary to see how well you are doing. You'll probably find that your sense of control builds with each experiment. Remember, you are creating accountability for yourself.

Another way of tracking successes in your journal is to keep track of foods that you avoid. If you walk away from the doughnuts in the conference room at work and you were able to pass on your favorite dessert at your favorite restaurant, write down those successful moments!

Remember the following advice when indulging:

Savor every bite. Turn off the TV. Eat in the dining room. Light a candle or two. Look at your treat. Smell your treat. Notice every single bite. Notice the taste and texture of at least the first bite. This may feel unusual to you at first, but you will eventually get used to it. Over time, eating with distraction will feel as foreign to you as eating without it may feel now.

If you find you resist focusing on your treat, think about why. Are you consciously tuning out to avoid feeling guilty about eating? In other words, do you tell yourself, "The calories don't count if I don't remember eating them"? Eating without distraction may take a little getting used to, but you'll eventually find that it increases the joy of eating and decreases your risk of overeating.

Find comfort by enriching your life. Many of the indulgence foods on the Level 2 menus are considered comfort foods. To ensure you stay in control as you eat these foods, it's essential that you find comfort in nonfood-related ways. You cannot use food to fill the emotional emptiness inside of you. You must enrich your life personally or professionally. Face the emptiness. Are you lonely? Then perhaps you need to develop closer friendships or speak with someone who can help you uncover the reasons why food has become one of your friends. Are you stressed? Find another outlet, such as deep breathing or walking. Are you angry? Face the problem that is making you feel that way and try to solve it.

WHAT TO EAT ON LEVEL 2

Level 2 brings you more food variety and fun. We've expanded your daily repertoire of foods to include a greater amount and variety of fruit, vegetables, starch, and more. Overall, you'll have more carbohydrates every day, eating somewhere between 51 and 150 grams.

If you are moving from Level 1 to Level 2, do so in steps. Don't suddenly go from eating 50 grams of carbohydrates to 150. That sudden jump can cause fatigue, hunger, and, possibly, a weight-loss plateau. Instead, slowly increase your consumption of carbohydrates by adding one carbohydrate serving a week, cutting back on 2 teaspoons of fat as you do so. Use the chart beginning on the opposite page to guide you in this quest. For example, during your first week at Level 2, you might add an extra serving of fruit (you only got one serving in Level 1; now you have two). On week 2, you might add oatmeal. On week three, an indulgence food. If at any time you notice you feel hungrier or more tired than usual, back off. That's a sign that your body is not yet ready for the increase in carbohydrates.

The basic menu that follows includes up to 150 grams of carbs. Keep in mind that you might not be able to consume the full 150 grams and still continue to lose weight. You might have to back off to 125 or 100 grams. That's why we've included the carbohydrate gram amounts for each category of food—so you can get an idea of how much you are adding or subtracting at any one time.

Follow this advice:

Keep tabs on your hunger and cravings. Every dieter transitions to Level 2 eating a little differently. Some people simply can't incorporate certain indulgence foods into their daily repertoire without going overboard. If you continually find that you lose control when you dish up ice cream or snack chips, then you may need to limit or eliminate these foods from your diet for a while and then try again a few months later. Incorporate only those indulgence foods that you can savor, eat guiltlessly, and stay in control of.

Pair carbs with fat and protein. This important guideline from Level 1 is even more important now that you'll be adding in more luxuries. (We'll give specific suggestions, starting on page 134.) Consume fruit only in conjunction with protein and fat to limit its effect on blood sugar. For example, have it with whipped cream, ricotta cheese, cottage cheese, or almond or peanut butter.

Indulge without guilt. No matter what your favorite indulgence foods are we've done the math for you, so you'll be consuming a balanced amount of carbohydrates that is designed to allow you to continue to lose weight. We've removed the guilt from your guilty pleasures!

LEVEL 2 DAILY PLAN

EAT THIS DAILY	VARIETIES	SERVING SIZES/DAY	CARBOHYDRATES PER SERVING
Protein foods	Beef Eggs Fish and shellfish (see page 54 for low-mercury varieties) Lamb Nitrate-free deli meat Nitrate-free sausages and franks Pork Poultry Tofu Wild game: bison, ostrich, venison	4 oz at breakfast (1 egg = 2 oz) 4 to 8 oz at lunch and dinner (3 oz meat, poultry, or fish = size of a deck of cards) 2 oz for snacks	0 g per oz
Leafy and green vegetables	Arugula Beet greens Bok choy Broccoli rabe Butterhead lettuce Celery Chard Collards Cucumber Endive Escarole Kale Mizuna Mustard greens Radicchio Red leaf lettuce Romaine Shallots Sorrel Spinach Turnip greens Watercress	3 to 5 cups raw (1 cup = 4 lettuce leaves)	1 g per cup

EAT THIS DAILY	VARIETIES	SERVING SIZES/DAY	CARBOHYDRATES PER SERVING
Vegetables	Artichoke Asparagus Bell peppers Broccoli Brussels sprouts Cabbage Cauliflower Chicory Eggplant Garlic Kohlrabi Leeks Onions Tomato Zucchini	1 cup raw vegetables OR 4 oz tomato or vegetable juice + ½ cup raw vegetables	7 to 15 g per cup
Starchy vegetables, legumes, pasta, rice, or oatmeal	Beans Corn Lentils Peas Pumpkin Rice, brown or wild Sweet potato Winter squash Whole grain pasta Steel-cut oats	½ cup cooked pasta or starch ¼ to ½ cup dry oatmeal	30 g
Fruit	Apple Apricots (8 medium) Blackberries Blueberries (1 cup) Canatloupe (¼ large) Cherries (40 medium) Grapefruit (1) Orange Peach Pear Pineapple fresh (1 cup diced) Plum Raspberries Strawberries Watermelon	2 small whole fruits or 1½ cups berries or diced fruit	15 g per oz

EAT THIS DAILY	VARIETIES	SERVING SIZES/DAY	CARBOHYDRATES PER SERVING
Dairy foods	Almond milk, unsweetened (½ cup) Any sliced or stick cheese (1 stick or 1 slice) Cottage cheese (¼ cup) Cream (1 oz) Cream cheese (1 Tbsp) Greek yogurt (½ cup) Ricotta cheese (¼ cup)	3 to 4 oz	½ cup or 1 g per oz
Bread	Recommended brands of bread and crackers (see page 94)*	2 slices bread or 2 crackers	15 g
Snacks	Avocado, 1 small Nuts, all varieties Olives, all varieties (28) Seeds, all varieties	2 oz nuts (2 oz = 46 whole almonds, 38 pecan halves, 2 Tbsp flaxseed, 2 Tbsp peanut or almond butter)	5 g per oz
Added fats	**For salad dressing:** Olive oil or recommended dressings (see page 95) **For cooking and spreads:** Butter unsalted Coconut oil Ghee Grapeseed oil High-heat cooking oil Mayonnaise Walnut oil	1½ to 3 Tbsp	0 g per Tbsp
Toppings and flavorings	Coconut, unsweetened and additive-free Condiments, unsweetened and additive-free, such as mustard, horse-radish, caponata, bruschetta Lemon or lime juice	2 oz lemon or lime juice ½ cup coconut	1 to 5 g per oz
Indulgence food	See information starting on page 134		15 to 30 g

* For the Ezekiel 4:9 bread, please note that 1-ounce serving is 1 slice.

INDULGE IN LUXURY FOODS

We want you on this plan for life, because we want to *save* your life. And we know the key to eating well long term is that you *enjoy* your life. So pick your plan, plan your indulgence, and get on with living! You may stick with just one plan or alternate among all of them. It's up to you.

If you tend to overeat sweet foods, you should probably not plan to consume desserts more than three or four times a week. This will allow you to practice your planning skills by exercising self-control.

If You Love Ice Cream

Because ice cream is high in sugar and low in overall nutrition, we recommend you have it no more than once a week at first. Eat it after dinner, when you have fewer hours to lose control and allow one serving to turn into two, three, or four. Choose any natural variety that does not contain additives, such as Breyer's or Julie's organic. Cream, sugar, and milk should be the only ingredients listed on the label. Carefully measure a ½-cup serving into a bowl (not a cone). You may use one of your daily fruit and/or nut servings as part of your ice cream indulgence by mixing these ingredients into the ice cream (à la Cold Stone Creamery) or sprinkling them on top.

If you continue to lose slowly, you can experiment with increasing your ice cream indulgence to twice and then three times a week. Again, pay careful attention to your cravings and your level of control. If you find yourself scooping spoonfuls straight out of the container, back off to just once a week or less often, perhaps just once every two weeks.

If You Crave Carbs

Yes, you can eat carbs and starch and still lose weight. Although the overall program aims to minimize starch, some people feel this reduction as a huge void in their lives. Our rule? Consume only high-quality starch, in the recommended portions, a few times a week. We want you to indulge your starch lust with whole grain and high-fiber options. Consult the "Fiber Scores" chart on page 99 to choose the highest-fiber starch options from various categories of foods. Always, always use starch as an accompaniment to a meal—that is, as a side dish—and not as the main attraction. Measure starch servings very carefully; don't eyeball them. One serving equals:

½ cup dry oatmeal

1 slice approved bread

1 approved cracker

½ cup cooked whole grain or fiber-fortified pasta

½ cup cooked beans/legumes

⅓ cup cooked brown or wild rice

1 small potato or ½ large potato

½ cup mashed sweet potato or yam

If You Need Salty Snacks

"No one can eat just one" is such an apt slogan for a potato chip. Once a week, you may have a single 1-ounce serving of any trans fats–free snack, such as pretzels or baked potato chips. (Check the list of ingredients to make sure the word *hydrogenated* does not appear. Packaged foods can claim they have zero trans fats even if they have up to 0.5 gram per serving.) Always consume salty snacks with a little fat to slow digestion and help you stay in control. Have them with 1 to 2 tablespoons of peanut or almond butter, avocado, ricotta cheese, or hummus.

If You Indulge in Beer and Wine

Instead of Happy Hour, go for after-dinner drinks. Hold yourself to one glass (12 ounces of beer, 5 ounces of wine, or 1½ ounces of hard liquor) and consume it with or at the end of the meal to reduce the chance of alcohol-induced munchies. Consume alcohol only once or twice a week. Consuming it every day may slow weight loss.

If You Love Chocolate

If you consume dark chocolate with an 85 percent or higher cocoa content, you may eat up to four squares a day (the suggested serving size on a package, or 40 grams). We've actually measured the blood sugar rise in patients after consuming this type of chocolate and have found that this luxury food is so high in fiber and so low in sugar that it hardly affects blood sugar at all. If you prefer sweeter chocolate (less cocoa, more sugar), substitute the same amount for a serving of starchy vegetables, pasta, or oatmeal to account for more sugar in the chocolate.

If, after adding chocolate, your cravings intensify or your weight loss slows, omit one serving of dairy food plus one serving of starchy vegetables, pasta, or oatmeal to get the scale moving in the right direction again.

SAMPLE MEAL PLANS

Use these meal plans to guide your eating choices. Feel free to mix and match various meals to create your own customized plans, or just use these as inspiration. Whenever possible, try to use our recommended brands (see page 94).

DAY 1

MORNING SNACK

4 celery sticks with 2 tablespoons peanut butter

Michelle's Relaxing Mocktail (page 230)

BRUNCH

Spinach and Feta Omelet (page 228)

2 turkey franks

7 large olives

Unsweetened iced tea

SNACK

1 small apple, sliced, with 1 ounce goat cheese melted on top

DINNER

Romaine salad made with:

- 3 cups romaine lettuce
- 1 ounce red bell pepper
- 1 ounce walnuts
- ½ avocado, sliced
- 1 tablespoon olive oil
- ½ tablespoon lemon juice
- 8 ounces cooked chicken, cubed
- ½ cup cooked broccoli
- ½ cup cooked carrots

Ice Cream Float (page 241)

DAY 2

BREAKFAST

Vanilla Almond Smoothie (page 228)

SNACK

1 turkey frank with 1 tablespoon mustard, 1 ounce sauerkraut, 1 whole grain hot dog bun

LUNCH

Cobb salad made with:
- 2 cups romaine lettuce
- 6 ounces sliced turkey
- 1 ounce sliced ham
- ¼ avocado, sliced
- 2 tomato wedges
- 1 tablespoons Caesar dressing

SNACK

2 roasted chicken drumsticks

1 tablespoon blue cheese dressing

DINNER

Soup made with:
- 1 cup beef broth
- 6 ounces broiled T-bone steak
- 3 cups bok choy, cooked in 1 teaspoon butter
- 5 ounces red wine

SNACK

3 ounces cottage cheese

1 small peach

DAY 3

BREAKFAST

Power Oatmeal (page 246)

2 ounces smoked salmon with ¼ avocado, 2 ounces diced cucumber

SNACK

3 celery sticks with 1 tablespoon almond butter

LUNCH

Salad made with:
- 1 cup lettuce
- ½ tablespoon olive oil
- 1 tablespoon lemon juice

Burger made with:
- 6 ounces cooked 85% lean ground beef
- 2 teaspoons mustard
- 1 tablespoon sautéed onion
- 1 ounce cooked portobello mushroom

2 slices Alvarado Street bread

SNACK

1 slice extra-firm tofu with:
- 1 ounce garlic and onion tomato sauce
- 1 ounce part-skim mozzarella cheese melted on top

DINNER

3 cups bok choy sautéed in ½ tablespoon coconut oil

Mexican Chicken Stir-Fry (page 240)

½ cup cooked brown rice

SNACK

½ cup whole strawberries with 1 tablespoon whipped cream

DAY 4

BREAKFAST

Eggs Florentine (page 229)

1 slice approved bread

SNACK

2 ounces Baked Cheese (page 235)

½ fresh pear

LUNCH

Salad made with:

- 3 cups romaine lettuce
- ½ cup mandarin oranges
- 2 tablespoons Caesar dressing

6 ounces sliced turkey with 1 tablespoon mustard

SNACK

½ avocado

3 ounces boiled shrimp with 1 teaspoon mayonnaise

1 ounce lightly salted kettle chips

DINNER

Chicken vegetable soup made with:

- 2 cups chicken broth
- ¼ cup cooked lentils
- ½ cup frozen garden vegetable stir-fry

Curry Chicken (page 240)

¼ cup green beans, cooked, mixed with ¼ cup bruschetta

SNACK

Roast beef roll-up made with:

- 2 ounces roast beef
- 2 ounces cheddar cheese
- 3 leaves red leaf lettuce

DAY 5

BREAKFAST

1 slice French Toast (page 227)

2 turkey franks

½ pink grapefruit

SNACK

3 celery sticks spread with 2 ounces tuna with 1 Tbsp mayonnaise

LUNCH

Grilled salmon kebobs made with:
- 6 ounces salmon
- 20 strips green bell pepper
- ½ cup cubed eggplant
- 1 garlic clove, minced and sprinkled over top

½ cup brown rice

SNACK

2 string cheese sticks

DINNER

Meatballs Florentine with Whole Grain Pasta (page 244)

Salad made with:
- 2 cups butterhead lettuce
- ¼ cup cherry tomatoes
- 1 tablespoon oil and vinegar dressing

SNACK

Ice Cream Float (page 241)

DAY 6

BREAKFAST

Ambrosia (page 246)

SNACK

Half a sandwich made with:
- 1 slice approved bread
- 3 ounces cooked chicken strips
- 1 tablespoon vinaigrette

LUNCH

Onion soup made with:
- 2 cups beef broth
- ¼ cup diced onion

Salad made with:
- 3 cups romaine lettuce
- 1 ounce olives
- 1 tablespoon Caesar dressing

4 ounces cooked London broil

½ medium sweet potato sprinkled with cinnamon

DINNER

6 ounces salmon encrusted with 1 tablespoon cooked flaxseed

2 cups collards cooked with 1 teaspoon butter

½ cup cooked spaghetti squash mixed with 1 teaspoon butter

SNACK

9 small oat bran pretzels dipped in one serving Red Pepper Hummus (page 242)

1 tablespoon almond butter

DAY 7

BREAKFAST

Turkey roll-up made with:
- 4 ounces sliced turkey breast
- 2 ounces cheese
- 4 leaves red leaf lettuce

SNACK

2 ounces cottage cheese

½ ounce walnuts

LUNCH

½ cup diced tomato

1 cup sliced cucumber dipped in 1 tablespoon ranch dressing

Mexican Meatloaf (page 245)

½ cup mandarin orange

DINNER

Shrimp salad made with:
- 6 large grilled shrimp
- ¼ cup sliced and peeled cucumber
- ½ cup boiled asparagus
- 3 cups spinach
- 2 tablespoons vinaigrette

SNACK

½ cup raspberries with 1 ounce whipped cream

2 squares 85% cacao dark chocolate

1 ounce almonds

1 cup decaf hazelnut coffee

RESTAURANT SUGGESTIONS

You have a little more leeway in Level 2, but don't allow your expanded menu options to unravel your sense of control. Stick mostly with the eating-out strategies from Level 1 (see page 123), but expand your options slightly. If you don't eat out very often, pick one way to indulge on Level 2. Most people overdo it. Instead of picking one luxury, they cheat for the entire meal. It starts with the bread basket, leads to a glass of wine or two, and ends with a huge serving of dessert. That's overdoing it, and if you overdo it like that, your weight loss will stall. You might treat yourself by having 1 roll before your meal, 1 alcoholic drink with your meal, ⅓ cup serving of starch, *or* splitting a dessert with your dining companions. It's your choice, but you must make a choice. You cannot have it all. Use the Food Lover's plans as basic guides for eating out.

MAINTENANCE IS AS EASY AS 1-2-3

Eating for life is very similar to eating for weight loss.

As you add in foods as suggested on the Level 2 chart (page 131), your weight loss will begin to slow. You will eventually plateau, and the point at which you plateau will vary. You might be able to increase your total carbohydrates to 60 to 80 grams before you plateau. You might be able to go up to 80 or 100. If you are very active, you might be able to consume as many as 150.

To find the right amount of carbohydrates for you, pay attention to the types and amounts of food you have added back, adding no more than one new food and serving a week. Once you plateau, you've reached your maintenance weight, also known as Level 3.

If you—oops—plateau before you've reached your goal, you may have added carbs back in too quickly. Slowly reduce your servings of carbs so that you start losing again, but not so many that you may feel deprived.

It bears repeating: Once you get to your goal weight, do not change your eating drastically. That's a recipe for regain! You'll eat this way for the rest of your life. Weigh yourself regularly and count carbs for a while, using the carb counts provided in the various food plans or any nutrition counter as a guide. Eventually, you'll get used to the basic repertoire of foods you can eat day in and day out, and you won't have to do so much counting when your new eating becomes a lifelong habit.

You've made a lot of changes in your diet. But one more step in your nutritional program will ensure your hard work takes full effect. Let's turn to Chapter 9 to add in your supplement prescription, a tailored plan that will make a big difference in your weight loss results as well as your energy, vitality, and long-term immunity.

THE SUPPLEMENT PRESCRIPTION

The supplements we recommend will help restore balance to your metabolic organs and hormone systems as you lose weight. This will improve your physical and mental well-being, helping you stick with your nutrition plan and eventually exercise.

We recommend seven supplements no matter your age, health, or weight-loss goal. Continue to take these supplements after you reach your goal. In addition to helping to heal the metabolism, they also promote good health. Long after you've dropped that final pound, these key supplements will help improve mood and energy levels, deepen sleep, and reduce your risk for heart disease, cancer, and osteoporosis.

If you have a specific metabolic disadvantage, we recommend that you take some of these key supplements in higher dosages. In some cases, we recommend additional supplements as well. Once you reach your weight loss goal and your health has improved, you can drop these dosages down to the standard dose.

MULTIVITAMIN/MINERAL

Look for: A supplement with 100 percent of the Daily Value (DV) of most vitamins and minerals, including iron, vitamin B$_{12}$, folic acid, magnesium, and vitamins A, E, and C.

Cautions: Depending on your health status or age, men and nonmenstruating women may not need to supplement iron; please consult your doctor. Many multivitamins contain soy and other binders. Read labels carefully.

You've probably heard that Americans are the most well nourished of the world's people. Although we may be well nourished in overall calories, most of us are malnourished when it comes to specific key nutrients. Various studies show, for example, that 95 percent of Americans are deficient in at least one nutrient. Common deficiencies include:

Folic acid. When levels are low, the risk of heart disease, birth defects, and breast cancer goes up.

Vitamin D. When levels are low, bones weaken. (More on vitamin D on the following pages.)

Antioxidant vitamins A, E, and C. Low levels increase the risk for heart disease, cancer, and several chronic diseases.

Malnourishment stems from three factors. First, many Americans consume the bulk of their calories from processed foods rather than from nutrient-packed foods such as fruits and vegetables. The average

YOUR SUPPLEMENT BUYING GUIDE

Purchase all supplements from companies with a GMP (Good Manufacturing Practice) seal. Read the list of ingredients to make sure the supplement does not use binders such as cornstarch. Most capsules contain soy lecithin, which is nearly inescapable. If you have a hormone disadvantage, consider taking liquid supplements or those from the brands Puritan's Pride or Solgar, or any other brand that has a GMP seal, most of which do not use soy as a binder. These are "must-haves" listed in order of importance:

1. Multivitamin/mineral—100 percent of the Daily Value (DV) for vitamins and minerals
2. Omega-3 fatty acids—1000 mg
3. Calcium (500 mg), magnesium (250 mg), boron (6 mg), and vitamin D (800 IU), either as separate supplements or as one or two combination capsules
4. Coenzyme Q10 (CoQ10)—30 mg
5. L-Carnitine—500 mg
6. Alpha-lipoic acid—100 mg
7. Probiotic—1 billion+ CFUs (colony-forming units)

American consumes only one and a half servings of vegetables, one serving of fruit, and one or fewer servings of whole grains each day. The vegetable serving often comes in the form of ketchup or french fries.

Second, our ability to absorb some nutrients—particularly B_{12} (critical for nerve function), magnesium (vital for muscles and nerves), and iron (an important component of red blood cells)—declines with age. Our ability to make vitamin D has declined due to the widespread (and good) use of sunscreen.

Third, food is less nutritious than in years past. When investigative health journalist Alex Jack analyzed data from the 2004 U.S. Department of Agriculture's National Nutrient Database and compared it with data from nutrient records from 1975, he came to a startling conclusion: Our fruits and vegetables are losing their nutrients. Broccoli, for example, had 50 percent less calcium than it did in the 1970s. Watercress had 88 percent less iron, cauliflower 40 percent less vitamin C, bell peppers 30 percent less vitamin C, apples 41 percent less vitamin A, and collards 57 percent less potassium. Why are these fuits and vegetables becoming less nutrient packed? The USDA has claimed that differences in testing techniques are to blame, but many experts have other explanations.

- According to research done at Iowa State University, the typical fruit or vegetable travels thousands of miles over several days to get from the farm where it was grown and harvested to the supermarket. Produce grown in Chile, Mexico, China, and other countries travels even farther. Levels of many vitamins and antioxidants drop as soon as a fruit or vegetable is picked. The longer it takes to go from stem to store, the less nutritious your produce. To ensure that some varieties of fruits and vegetables are not overripe when they reach the store, farmers pick them earlier in the ripening cycle. The less ripe a fruit or vegetable is at harvest, the fewer nutrients it will contain.
- Commercial fertilizers may cause fruits and vegetables to absorb more water, which dilutes their nutrient content and flavor.
- Biotechnology companies have developed seeds designed to produce supersized fruits and vegetables that naturally resist pests and molds. When they engineer these supergrowth qualities into the seeds, something else generally gets engineered out—and that something else is usually nutritional quality and flavor.
- Today our atmosphere contains more carbon dioxide than in years

past. This increased CO_2 causes plants to produce fruits and vegetables with greater amounts of starch. The higher the starch content of a vegetable, generally the lower the nutrient content. Carbon dioxide also leads to acid rain that demineralizes soil and the produce grown in that soil.

It's clear that you need a multivitamin. Just walk into any supplement store, however, and you can be easily overwhelmed by all of the different brands clamoring for your attention. Do you need a women's or a men's formula? Should you choose a stress formula? Is a whole food supplement better than other types?

We like to keep things simple. Look for a supplement with balanced amounts of the major vitamins and minerals. It should have at least 100 percent of the recommended Daily Values (DVs) for iron, vitamin B_{12}, folic acid, magnesium, and vitamins A, E, and C. This is the bare minimum needed to protect against deficiency. You'll need higher amounts of specific vitamins and minerals—particularly calcium, vitamin D, and magnesium—to protect against disease and bring your metabolism back into balance. That's why we've recommended purchasing those as separate supplements.

Regardless of your gender, stay away from "women's formulas." Many of these contain soy. Soy has made its way into so many foods that no one needs even more of it in a supplement. Believe us, you are already getting all of the soy you need from your bread, chocolate, and commercial hamburgers.

Coenzyme Q10 (CoQ10)

Look for: A supplement with 30 milligrams of CoQ10 in a fat-soluble form to be taken once a day, in the morning. If you feel fatigued, have heart disease, or have an insulin disadvantage, go up to 100 milligrams.

Cautions: Make sure your physician knows you plan to take this supplement. It can interact with some medications, particularly the blood thinner coumadin (Warfarin) and blood pressure drugs.

You're saying, "CoQ what?" If you've never heard of this supplement, it's the fault of the medical establishment, which has not yet caught on to the vast number of studies that show just how important it is to good health. CoQ10 is an antioxidant found in the membranes of our cells. It's no accident that it's concentrated in the cell mitochondria, or energy compartment. Just as your car creates air pollution when it burns gasoline to produce energy, your cells create pollution in the form of free radicals when they use oxygen and glucose to create adenosine triphosphate (ATP), the currency that the body recognizes as energy. CoQ10 neutralizes these free radicals, preventing them from damaging cells, tissues, proteins, and DNA. CoQ10 is also instrumental in a number of cell reactions. It's particularly important for heart health. Yet, most people over age 30 are low in CoQ10 for a number of reasons.

- Some prescription medicines reduce levels of CoQ10. They include: tricyclic antidepressants (Elavil and Tofranil), the antipsychotic drug Haloperidol, cholesterol-lowering statin drugs such as Lovastatin and Pravastatin, beta-blockers, antidiabetic sulfonylurea drugs such as Glucotrol and Micronase, and the anti-hypertension drug Clonidine. These common medications interfere with the body's synthesis of CoQ10 and may cause a deficiency of this crucial compound.
- CoQ10 is poorly absorbed.
- CoQ10 levels decrease with age. Depletion starts at age 20 and, by age 50, we have about 50 percent less of it.

Research shows that CoQ10 supplements can lower blood pressure, slow the development of dementia, improve exercise performance in people with heart disease, reduce gum disease, and increase sperm count. Supplemental CoQ10 may also reduce the incidence of migraines and lower cancer risk.

Omega-3 Fatty Acids

Look for: A supplement with 1,000 milligrams of combined alpha-linolenic acid (ALA), eicosapentaenoic acid (EPA), and docosahexaenoic acid (DHA). Take one in the morning.

Cautions: Tell your doctor before you take this supplement, especially if you bruise easily or are taking a blood-thinning medication such as Coumadin.

Most of us consume too many omega-6 fatty acids in the form of vegetable oils (mostly from processed foods made with vegetable oils) and too few omega-3 fats. Although both types of fats are healthy, too much omega-6 and too little omega-3 throws off the body's balance, triggering pro-inflammatory molecules to form. This raises risk for just about every disease of aging—and it also blocks weight loss.

In an ideal world, you would be able to consume all of the omega-3 fatty acids you need from food, but we do not live in an ideal world. Fish, the primary food source of these fats, is increasingly contaminated with mercury, dioxin, polychlorinated biphenyls (PCBs), and other carcinogens and toxins. These substances are present at low levels in fresh waters and oceans. They are present in the algae and other plant foods that the smallest fish eat. Because PCBs and mercury have long half-lives, they tend to become more concentrated in each progressive step up the food chain. They are generally highest in the older, longer-lived, predatory fish, but all fish, including anchovies and shrimp, contain some environmental contaminants.

Just as they accumulate in long-lived fish, these chemicals also accumulate in people, especially people who eat fish on a regular basis. A recent study done by the New York City Health Department, for example, revealed that one in four New Yorkers had elevated mercury levels. A similar survey shows that San Franciscans also have high levels of this neurotoxin.

It used to be that meat and eggs also supplied omega-3 fatty acids, but conventional farming practices are producing meat and eggs that are lower in this important fat.

This makes supplementation a must. By keeping omega-3s in balance with omega-6s, this supplement will help elevate your mood, improve metabolism, lower triglycerides, lower blood pressure, ease inflammatory skin conditions such as psoriasis and eczema, reduce menstrual cramping, and lower the risk of heart attack, dangerous abnormal heart rhythms, stroke, rheumatoid arthritis, and specific cancers.

But won't your supplement contain mercury and other contaminants? Probably not. Testing by ConsumerLab.com—an independent supplement testing company—determined that most fish oil supplements were free of mercury and other contaminants common to fish. The nonprofit group Environmental Defense (ED) has also done studies on supplement safety and has determined that two-thirds of polled companies follow strict procedures to limit environmental contaminants in their fish oil supplements.

Calcium with Magnesium, Boron, and Vitamin D

Look for: A supplement that contains calcium and magnesium in a 2 to 1 ratio (example: 1,000 milligrams of calcium and 500 milligrams of magnesium). Take at least once a day, preferably before bed to aid sleep. Take either a separate or combined supplement that also contains 800 IUs of vitamin D and 6 milligrams of boron.

Cautions: Calcium may interfere with thyroid medications, so do not take both at the same time. Choose calcium-mineral supplements carefully. A study published in the *Journal of the American Medical Association* determined that some calcium supplements, particularly the ones made from oyster shells, were contaminated with small amounts of lead. TriMedica is one brand that is 99.9 percent lead-free.

You've probably heard that calcium is important for strong bones, and it is. But did you know it can also stimulate weight loss? At least six studies to date have shown that women who consume more calcium—either through food or through supplements—tend to weigh less and have less body fat than women who consume less calcium. For example, when researchers supplemented overweight African-Americans with 1,000 daily milligrams of calcium, the women lost weight effortlessly. Multiple studies have been completed since and have continued to find the same beneficial results. People who consume more calcium—through supplements or food—tend to weigh less than people who don't. Dieters who take calcium lose more weight than dieters who do not.

Some experts have tried to explain away this connection, saying that women who consume more calcium tend to exercise and eat more healthfully than women who consume less, so it makes sense that they would weigh less, too. That may be true, but there are also many real mechanisms by which calcium may improve your fat-burning ability. Michael Zemel, PhD, a researcher at the University of Tennessee, for example, has shown that mice fed a low-calcium, low-calorie diet do not lose weight as quickly as mice fed a high-calcium, low-calorie diet. Lack of calcium seems to somehow impede fat burning. Calcium may help by turning up fat burning after a meal and switching off fat storage, Zemel has concluded.

Finally, research shows that low-calcium diets tend to turn off a fat-burning switch, whereas high-calcium intake turns that switch on.

Calcium may also stimulate the release of fat from fat cells—so it can be burned for energy—and block the development of new fat cells.

But calcium, studies show, works best when it's paired with vitamin D. This holds true for every benefit of calcium—it doesn't seem to effectively induce fat burning, build bones, or protect against cancer unless vitamin D comes along for the ride. Vitamin D helps your body absorb calcium, and it provides many additional health protective properties. Boron and magnesium are also important and seem to work in tandem with calcium. Magnesium, in particular, helps counteract the constipating effect of calcium, keeping you regular. When you take calcium, vitamin D, magnesium, and boron together, you will enhance weight loss and build stronger bones. Calcium has also been linked to the following benefits.

Cancer protection. Calcium and vitamin D have been shown to reduce colon cancer risk. In a 4-year study of more than 800 people, those who took calcium and vitamin D were less likely to develop benign tumors that tend to lead to cancer in the colon or rectum. Only people who took both calcium and vitamin D had this effect, however. Neither calcium nor vitamin D alone reduced risk.

Milder PMS. According to the long-term Nurse's Health Study of thousands of women, women who consumed the equivalent of 1,200 milligrams of calcium and 400 IUs of vitamin D were less likely to be diagnosed with PMS during the 10-year study than women who consumed less of either vitamin or mineral. (Magnesium is also important for PMS.)

Lower blood pressure. Magnesium helps regulate blood pressure, and people who consume more magnesium through food or supplements tend to see a drop in pressure.

Reduced risk of diabetes. The body needs magnesium to process carbohydrates and fats and to produce energy.

A longer life. Studies show that people who take vitamin D supplements have a lower risk of death from all causes. Based on research results of 18 different studies, researchers determined that deficiencies in vitamin D raised the risk of death from cancer, heart disease, and diabetes. Based on this research, people who took vitamin D had a 7 percent lower risk of death than those who did not.

You've probably heard that you can consume calcium through dairy products, fish, and fortified foods. Why supplement? As it turns out, dairy and fortified foods may not be the best way to get your calcium, for the following reasons:

- We don't want you drinking any milk on this plan due to its high sugar content. This sugar, called lactose, also tends to cause gas, bloating, and cramping in the vast majority of adults because their intestines no longer have the enzyme needed to break it down. In women, high levels of galactose, a sugar released when we digest lactose, may damage the ovaries, leading to ovarian cancer. In men, milk may also raise the risk for prostate cancer. In a large study of thousands of men conducted by Harvard researchers, men who drank two or more glasses of milk a day were almost twice as likely to develop advanced prostate cancer as those who didn't drink milk.

- Although food manufacturers have fortified many cereals, orange juice, and a few other processed foods with the equivalent of a calcium supplement, nearly all of these foods are high in carbohydrates. Because you will be restricting them, they are not the best way to get your calcium. Also, research completed at Creighton University in Omaha, Nebraska, shows that the body does not absorb calcium as well from many fortified products as it does from a supplement.

One of the reasons we recommend you eat so many greens and vegetables on this plan is because these foods are rich in calcium. (They're also packed with fiber, vitamins, antioxidants, and overall great nutrition.) But you need to supplement to ensure you get plenty of calcium.

L-Carnitine

Look for: A supplement with 500 milligrams of L-carnitine. Take it on an empty stomach before meals.

Cautions: None.

L-carnitine is made in the body from the amino acid lysine, is found in nearly every cell in the body, and is a critical player in energy production, literally carrying fat into the cells' mitochondria, where it is burned for energy. L-carnitine is also an antioxidant that protects cells against damage from free radicals. You probably need more L-carnitine as you age; tests done on seniors have shown that L-carnitine levels decline with age, and supplements reverse this decline.

Alpha-Lipoic Acid (ALA)

Look for: A supplement with 100 milligrams of alpha-lipoic acid. Take it on an empty stomach before meals up to three times a day.

Cautions: None.

Alpha-lipoic acid, like L-carnitine, is produced by the body and is involved in energy production. It also functions as a strong antioxidant and helps stabilize blood glucose.

When researchers supplemented old rats with alpha-lipoic acid, their mitochondria, the fat-burning furnaces of their cells, functioned better and produced fewer age-promoting free radicals. The rats also experienced a boost in memory. When rats were supplemented with both L-carnitine (mentioned earlier) and alpha-lipoic acid, mitochondrial function improved even more.

Probiotic

Look for: Jarrow, Solgar, Nature's Way, and other brands. Your brand should have at least 1 billion bacteria, especially the lactobacillus type.

Cautions: None.

You don't need to have a yeast disadvantage to benefit from a probiotic supplement. In our opinion, everyone should take one. We even recommend them for children.

A probiotic supplement introduces good bacteria into your GI tract. The word *probiotic* means "for life." These healthy types of bacteria have been shown to improve weight loss, bolster immunity, reduce the risk of certain cancers, improve bowel health, synthesize nutrients, and reduce allergy symptoms. They may improve blood sugar control by preventing the absorption of sugar into the bloodstream. They may promote weight loss by keeping yeast and certain types of bacteria in check, preventing these organisms from releasing toxins that slow the metabolism.

Broad-spectrum antibiotics such as tetracycline and ciprofloxacin kill both good and bad bacteria, allowing bad bacteria and yeast to proliferate. A high-sugar diet or use of birth control pills may contribute to yeast overgrowth and good bacteria undergrowth.

Your probiotic supplement will help restore a healthy balance to your digestive tract. This will help calm gas and bloating and will provide some side benefits. Men and women who took a probiotic bacteria supplement during the 2 weeks before and after getting a flu shot had a better immune response and were less likely to develop the flu in the following 5 months compared to people who did not take a probiotic supplement. In another study of 477 people, those who took a probiotic and a multivitamin for 3 months during the winter were 13 percent less likely to get sick than others who did not take the supplements.

SUPPLEMENT PLANS FOR METABOLIC DISADVANTAGE TYPES

In addition to the "must-have" list of supplements, you'll need a few others if you have a metabolic disadvantage (see Chapter 5).

Insulin Disadvantage

Alpha-Lipoic Acid (300 mg): The dose of alpha-lipoic acid (ALA) we recommended for everyone is too low for you. You need more ALA to reduce the side effects of high insulin levels. A study done at the Mayo Clinic and a medical center in Russia found that supplemental alpha-lipoic acid significantly reduced the frequency and severity of diabetic neuropathy symptoms such as burning, pain, prickling sensations, and numbness.

Biotin (3 mg): Biotin is a water-soluble B vitamin that can only be synthesized by bacteria, yeasts, molds, algae, and some plants. People with diabetes tend to be low in this vitamin. In one study, people with diabetes who had lower fasting blood glucose levels had higher blood biotin levels. In another study, people with diabetes who took 9 milligrams of biotin daily for a month experienced a 45 percent drop in fasting blood glucose levels. As a side benefit, it may also strengthen your fingernails.

Cinnamon (1 g): At least two studies have linked the spice cinnamon with reduced blood glucose, triglycerides, and LDL cholesterol in people with type 2 diabetes. In one of these studies, completed in Pakistan, 60 people with type 2 diabetes were divided into six groups of 10. Three groups took cinnamon capsules ranging in strength from 1 to 6 grams of cinnamon a day. The other three groups took placebo capsules. Everyone in the cinnamon group improved their blood sugar control, regardless of the strength of the capsules.

L-carnitine (1,000 mg): If you have an insulin disadvantage, high insulin levels are encouraging your body to hold on to fat. Because L-carnitine increases fat metabolism, it's particularly important for anyone with an insulin disadvantage. It may also improve testosterone levels in men.

Chromium (200 mcg of a "GTF" or chelated type): This mineral enhances the effects of insulin, helping the hormone do its job more easily. When insulin does its job better, the pancreas makes lower amounts of insulin, so levels stay lower. Low insulin keeps your energy levels steady, reduces hunger, and prompts your body to burn fat rather than store it. Studies show that chromium supplementation improves insulin function, glucose tolerance, and blood sugar control. If you've been eating a diet high in sugar (either from sugarcane or high-fructose corn syrup), you're probably low in this mineral. Sugar encourages the body to excrete chromium in the urine, decreasing levels of the mineral.

Yeast Disadvantage

Caprylic acid (650 mg), oil of oregano (600 mg), or olive leaf extract (500 mg): These are all natural antifungals that help reduce levels of yeast in the digestive tract. They are sold at health food stores in capsule form. Start with a half dose of one of these (325 mg of caprylic acid, 300 mg of oil of oregano, or 250 mg of olive leaf extract) and slowly work your way up to a full dose. Starting with the full dose too quickly causes an overly fast yeast die-off, and you may experience uncomfortable flulike symptoms from detoxing too quickly. Once your gas and bloating resolve, discontinue use.

Vitamin C (1,000 mg of Ester-C): This vitamin helps strengthen your immune system, so it's better able to reduce yeast levels.

Thyroid Disadvantage

Selenium (100 mcg): This antioxidant trace mineral has been shown to reduce the inflammation that can lead to thyroid dysfunction.

Zinc (30 mg): This is another mineral that is involved in thyroid function and is crucial for the production of thyroid hormone. If you are deficient in zinc, your thyroid hormone will drop and so will your metabolic rate. One study shows that zinc supplementation helps bolster levels of thyroid hormone and speeds metabolic rate.

Hormone Disadvantage

CoQ10 (100 mg): We included CoQ10 in the list of supplements that everyone should take because it is so important to overall health. It's even more important if you have a hormone disadvantage, which is why the dosage is higher.

L-carnitine (500 mg): You need a higher dose of this supplement to balance hormone levels and improve digestion and use of fat.

Calcium (1,000 mg) and magnesium (500 mg): We included calcium and magnesium in the list of supplements that everyone should take, but increase the dosage if you have a hormone disadvantage.

Adrenal Disadvantage

B complex (50 mg): When cortisol levels rise and stay elevated, our cells have a harder time defending themselves against the free radicals that are formed during everyday metabolic processes. When you are under stress, more free radicals form, depleting the body's natural abilities to neutralize them. That's where B complex vitamins come in. They protect cells from free radical damage. They also boost immunity, which so often erodes during times of stress.

CoQ10 (100 mg): We included CoQ10 in the list of supplements that everyone should take because it is so important to overall health. It's even more important if you have chronically high cortisol levels, because this antioxidant protects the body against oxidative stress. So for you, we've upped the dose.

You now have your entire nutritional plan mapped out. What's left, you ask? Oh, just what you do the other 20 hours of your day: how you make a living, how you manage your stress, and most important, how you recharge. Let's learn more about why rest is so critical to weight loss—and why you and your body deserve some more peace and quiet, starting tonight.

THE REST PRESCRIPTION

Now you know how to eat and which supplements to take. You might be thinking, "Okay, I'm ready to get started. Let's skip this chapter. What does rest have to do with weight loss?"

We're so glad you asked, because rest has *everything* to do with weight loss. Chronic unrest—lack of sleep coupled with a high-stress lifestyle—can nullify the best diet and supplement plan. We've seen this happen so often in practice. We counsel a patient who seems to be doing everything right. According to her food records, she's eating exactly as prescribed, yet the weight isn't budging. Then we dig a little deeper and learn that she's up repeatedly at night to soothe her kids back to sleep, on the go constantly during the day, and draining herself further with intense exercise at the gym.

This type of unrest keeps the fight-or-flight response in a permanent "on" position. Our bodies are designed to handle periodic influxes of stress hormones. Triggering your flight or fight response just once a day probably won't interfere with weight loss, because your body easily clears these hormones. Triggering it every 5 minutes? That's a recipe for weight gain.

Here's why. Every time you trigger your stress response, your adrenal glands pump out the stress hormone cortisol. If cortisol levels remain high—as they do when you don't get enough sleep, keep yourself awake during the day by consuming lots of caffeine, or generally feel edgy and jittery—your entire metabolism becomes imbalanced, suppressing thyroid function, raising blood sugar and blood pressure, weakening muscles and bones, and triggering the body to store more abdominal fat.

That's right: If you deal with stress poorly, allowing life to rev you up and agitate you, you'll see the results on your waistline. Consider:

- A study of 45,810 people determined that those who indicated greater amounts of job strain were more likely to be heavy than those who indicated lesser amounts of strain.
- Parents of children with cancer tend to gain more weight than parents of healthy kids, even though the former consume *fewer* calories.
- In a study of 225 British men and women, people who responded to challenging tasks with increased heart rates, blood pressure, and other stress indictors tended to be heavier than people who responded more calmly to these mental challenges.
- Various studies done on rats and humans show that stress hormones encourage us to do one of three things: exercise (in a rat's case, run on a wheel), eat (usually comfort foods that are high in sugar and fat, such as most desserts), or self-medicate (drink a beer, in the case of humans). This is why chronic stress tends to erode the willpower you need to follow a meal plan.

When you react poorly to stress, cortisol remains high when it should be low. Elevated cortisol causes blood sugar and insulin to rise, which directs extra calories into abdominal fat cells. Stress also causes you to crave carbs, as they chemically can make you feel relaxed by helping your brain make the calming neurochemical serotonin. This, over time, depletes serotonin levels, causing deficiency.

To lose weight and keep it off, you need to stop the cycle. Rather than constantly taxing your adrenal glands, you need to allow them time to rest and rebuild. When you allow cortisol levels to return to

EVEN WORSE THAN WEIGHT GAIN . . .

Stress has been linked with heart disease, stroke, cancer, and chronic lower respiratory diseases. It worsens asthma, rheumatoid arthritis, and gastrointestinal problems.

normal, your body will stop stockpiling fat in your abdomen. Your cravings for sweets will also diminish, and you'll develop the consistent energy you will need to exercise.

How do you rest the adrenals? The answer differs from person to person. Your specific rest prescription depends on two variables.

1. **The lifestyle habits you are willing to change**

2. **The extent of the problem**

You probably already know what you are willing and not willing to do. Keith, for instance, doesn't need to take a quiz or answer a series of self-reflective questions to know that he is not willing to take a meditation class. But he's willing to relax in many other ways, including taking a short walk after work to give himself some quiet time before entering a home environment that includes three young children. You'll find a number of stress-reduction techniques and activities in this chapter. Use whichever techniques make sense to you.

Now, let's determine the extent of your problem. We all have stress. We all can benefit from reducing stress, improving sleep, and relaxing more. Just how diligently you must work to reduce stress, however, depends on how intensely and how often you tend to trigger your stress response. To gauge these factors, answer yes or no to each of the following questions.

1. Do you sleep fewer than 7 hours at night?

☐ YES   ☐ NO

2. Do you take part in endurance exercise (such as marathoning or long-distance cycling) or power lifting?

☐ YES   ☐ NO

3. Do you feel on edge most of the time?

☐ YES   ☐ NO

4. Do you feel as if you don't have time to make love to your partner?

☐ YES   ☐ NO

5. Do you feel restless?

☐ YES   ☐ NO

6. Do you keep yourself going with caffeine or food?

☐ YES   ☐ NO

7. Do you work every day, including weekends?

☐ YES   ☐ NO

8. Do you feel achy for unexplainable reasons?

☐ YES   ☐ NO

9. Do you feel as if getting through each day is a matter of surviving from one moment to the next?

☐ YES   ☐ NO

10. Do you feel guilty when you take time for yourself?

☐ YES   ☐ NO

11. When you try to relax, do you feel anxious, as if you should be doing something more productive?

☐ YES   ☐ NO

12. Do you drink alcohol or eat sweets before bedtime?

☐ YES   ☐ NO

13. Do you wake because your spouse snores, pets disturb you, or small children summon you?

☐ YES   ☐ NO

14. Does it take you longer than 30 minutes to fall asleep?

☐ YES   ☐ NO

15. Do you feel tired when you wake in the morning?

☐ YES   ☐ NO

16. Do you feel drowsy during the day?

☐ YES   ☐ NO

Your number of "yes" answers: _____

Unless you're reading this book in a monastery high in the Himalayas, you have stress in your life. We all do. We all get stuck in traffic from time to time. We all must stand in long lines. Most of us have too much on our to-do lists to actually accomplish in a given day. We all have bills to pay, food shopping to do, meals to cook, and many other potentially stressful daily events.

The difference between someone with high cortisol and someone with low cortisol isn't in the number or magnitude of the stressors, it's in the response to them. If you answered yes to two or fewer questions, you are a low stress responder. The coping strategies under the heading "Daily Habits" below may be all you need. If you answered yes to three or more questions, you are a high stress responder. That means you not only have a high level of stress in your life, but you also have few coping mechanisms. In addition to incorporating the daily habits into your life, it's probably also a good idea to make daily use of one of the formal practices (see page 164), at least until you feel calmer and your sleep improves.

Keep in mind that only you are in control of your stress.

HOW TO DE-STRESS

We recommend you get in the habit of noticing your level of stress once a day. Monitor it on a scale of 1 to 10, with 1 being asleep and 10 being a life or death emergency. We all need some stress to function, so don't expect your ratings to stay below 2 day after day. If you were that calm, you might not find the motivation to get out of bed! On the other hand, if you feel stress that reaches above a 5 on a regular basis, you may need to take some additional stress-reducing precautions. Let's talk about some possibilities.

DAILY HABITS

If you have daily ways of recharging your emotional and physical batteries, you will be better able to weather the tough times during your weight loss journey. Choose from the following list of stress reducers.

Periodically, every day: Take a break from whatever you are doing to de-stress. You might take a short walk around the block, call a friend, play catch or tug-of-war with your dog, or find something funny to watch on YouTube. On a break at work, scope out a bench outside facing something green, even if it's just a small tree. Try the following breathing technique several times a day: Put both hands on your tummy and feel your tummy expand with each inhalation and contract with each exhalation. Pay attention to your breath like this for 1 minute.

On the way to work: If you commute by train or bus, don't read the paper. It's just an added source of stress. Instead, read a novel, sleep, breathe deeply, or listen to relaxing music. Look out the window and let your thoughts wander—this "idle" time allows your brain to reboot and be recharged and ready when you get to your desk. If you commute by car, minimize your exposure to depressing news or shock radio— instead, listen to books on CD or from your MP3 player.

At every meal: Eat mindfully in a calm environment. Allow your meals to serve as short, calm moments in an otherwise busy day. If the cafeteria at work is too loud or filled with people you don't want to talk to, take your lunch and find a table outside or in a quiet conference room or sitting area. Try not to eat in front of your computer, while driving, or while watching TV. These distractions reduce your perception of the taste, texture, and aroma of the food you are eating, causing you to feel unsatisfied after you finish everything on your plate. They also trigger the stress response, which can result in indigestion. Instead, make your meal calm and enjoyable. Before diving in, take a moment to center yourself. Then notice the colors, texture, smell, and taste of each bite. Chew thoroughly and take your time.

After work: Create a 5- to 10-minute buffer between the end of the workday and the beginning of the family circus. Turn off your BlackBerry and cell phone. Go for a walk, sit quietly, or listen to one or two of your favorite songs.

Get out of the house: Have you ever noticed that you sleep better and feel happier when you have a busy social calendar? That's because engaging socially helps your body relax. The vagus nerve—which connects the brain stem to the heart, lungs, and intestines—slows heart rate, lowers blood pressure, and calms the body. Part of this nerve, called the myelinated vagus, links the brain nerves to the face, allowing facial expressions to influence stress response. When you tune in to social cues—the smiles and laughter of your friends—these nerves send calming signals through your body.

FORMAL PRACTICES

If you feel very tense most of the day, every day, you may be out of touch with what it feels like to be relaxed. Stress, thankfully, is not a terminal illness. You can retrain your body to relax. Once a day, for 10 to 20 minutes, try any of the following relaxation techniques. Once you become adept at the techniques, you can use them for a shorter period of time and less often to maintain their calming effects.

Breath meditation: Sit quietly. Close your eyes. Breathe slowly. As you inhale, mentally say "one" to yourself. As you exhale, say "two." Inhale to "three." Exhale to "four." Do this up to five, and then breathe back down to one and start over again. Once you become adept at using breath counting to calm yourself, you will be able to quickly use the technique to reach a state of calm and focus when you feel stressed during the day.

Body scan: Sit comfortably or lie on your back. Close your eyes and breathe for a few seconds. Then bring your awareness to the sensations you feel in your face. Explore how your eye sockets feel. Move along to your cheeks and forehead. Notice your scalp. Do not judge how it feels. Just notice, as if you are exploring your body. There's also no need to physically try to relax. As you bring your awareness inward, your body will automatically relax. Continue to explore your entire head, then move down the body, starting with your neck, your chest, your shoulders, your right arm, your left arm, your abdomen, and so on, until you've reached your feet.

Self-awareness: Sit comfortably or lie on your back. Close your eyes and breathe for a few seconds. Bring your awareness to your thoughts. Notice the thoughts running through your mind. Then bring your awareness to your emotions. Do you feel angry? Happy? Tense? Scared? Then notice your body sensations. Do you have muscular tension? Are you hot or cold? Is your mouth dry or just right? Make no effort to change what you notice or to try to relax. The relaxation will come automatically.

Yoga: Take a class or use a video. Tai chi and Pilates are great, too.

WHY EXERCISE DOESN'T DE-STRESS

Many people claim to run away stress on the treadmill or beat it out in a kickboxing class. Yet, exercise is buying into the fight-or-flight response. This provides an outlet for the cortisol, so you use it. But it doesn't stop the stress response, so it can actually make things worse, quickening your journey to adrenal fatigue. Exercise stimulates the sympathetic nervous system, which interferes with the function of the vagus nerve, the main network the body uses to send calming signals to the heart and blood vessels. Exercise tells the body, "I'm running—I'm still in danger," reducing your relaxation response.

HOW TO IMPROVE SLEEP

Think about how well you sleep. If you routinely get less than 7 hours, wake more than once a night, or wake and find yourself unable to get back to sleep, you may need to put some effort into improving your sleep. Sleep is important, not only for your mental well-being but also for your waistline and health. Sleep restores the body. You need enough time to sleep, but more important, you need quality sleep. It needs to be a continuous, uninterrupted stretch that will allow you to fully cycle through all the stages of sleep, from Stage 1 (the lightest sleep) to Stage 4 (the deepest) to Stage 5 (rapid eye movement or REM), about five or six times during the night. Especially important are Stages 3 and 4, toward the beginning of your time in bed, during which you experience the most healing sleep—your blood pressure drops, breathing slows, and various hormones are released for restoration.

Studies have consistently linked poor sleep with increased body weight. The brain system that controls the sleep-wake cycle may also regulate appetite and metabolism. The hormone leptin rises during sleep, signaling a decrease in hunger. When you don't sleep, leptin stays low, and appetite stays high. Lack of sleep also raises the risk for developing diabetes, heart disease, and depression.

What's the right amount of sleep? There's no set number of hours that works for every single person. Most people probably need somewhere between 7 and 8 hours each night. If you are very sleep deprived, athletic, or recovering from illness, you may initially need more sleep. You may need 9 today to feel rested, but over time, after your metabolism repairs, you may do okay on 7 hours. If you do not feel rested when the alarm goes off, you are not getting enough deep sleep.

Consider the following questions. Do you:

- Take longer than 30 minutes to fall asleep at night?
- Wake more than once at night?
- Wake too early, long before your alarm rings and before you wish to get out of bed?
- Wake at night and have trouble getting back to sleep?

If you answered yes to any of those questions, you are sleep deprived. Your stress-reducing tactics, your supplement plan, and even your new eating habits will help improve your sleep. (For example, as your eating habits help normalize your blood glucose levels, you'll be less likely to wake between 1 and 4 a.m., when blood glucose is lowest.) To make sleep even more restful, try a few additional strategies.

Cut back on caffeine. As we mentioned earlier, it takes 3 to 7 hours for your body to eliminate half of the caffeine you've consumed. If you are taking oral contraceptives, it can take 5 to 10 hours. That's only half of the caffeine, which means that the other half is still in your body, disturbing sleep. If you drink coffee, tea, or other caffeinated beverages and you have disturbed sleep, try to eliminate them or at least confine your caffeine consumption to the morning hours.

Avoid drinking alcohol. Although alcohol may make you feel sleepy, it generally blocks you from getting into the deeper stages of sleep and makes you more likely to wake.

Dim the lights. Your brain has a circadian biological clock that directs your sleep-wake cycle. Called the suprachiasmatic nucleus (SCN), this part of the brain is influenced by light. For this reason, you tend to feel sleepy when it is dark and wake when it is light. Even the light from a television or computer screen, for example, seems to throw off the sleep-wake cycle, causing the brain to make less of the sleep-inducing hormone melatonin. Bright room lighting may also have this effect. Use these tips.

- Keep your bedroom as dark as possible. Use opaque shades on the windows. Cover or replace clocks that have bright digital displays, and get rid of the night-light.
- Install dimmers on your room and overhead light switches. About 30 to 60 minutes before bed, turn down the lights to signal to your brain that it's time to feel sleepy.
- Don't watch TV, work at the computer, or send text messages in the 15 minutes immediately before bedtime.

Eliminate distractions. Most people sleep better if they sleep alone. Kick the dog or cat off the bed. If your partner snores, invest in earplugs. If needed, sleep in a guest room, away from your partner.

Wind down. Most of us spend our days in "go" mode. With the brain constantly excited all day long, it's no wonder we struggle to wind down at night. Find a way to put a period—a rest—at the end of your day. Spend the last 15 minutes before bedtime calming yourself for bed. Don't do anything intellectually stimulating. Turn off your cell phone. Power down the computer. Take a shower. Put one book on your nightstand—no magazines or newspapers—and make it a boring one. Take a few minutes to jot down your thoughts or your plans for the next day in a journal. Many people find that these practices prevent middle-of-the-night insomnia due to fretful worries.

Use your bed only for sleep and sex. This will condition your mind that getting into bed is synonymous with falling asleep—after the sex, of course.

Try this supplement. Consider taking the herb valerian. A number of studies show that, when taken at bedtime, it improves sleep onset and duration. Take it either as a 300 milligram capsule or as a tea before bed. Just make sure your brand does not contain alcohol, as many do. Another supplement called inositol has been shown to enhance REM sleep. Take 100 milligrams before bed.

Now you're ready. You have all the tools you need to begin the full program, from your satisfying and incredibly healthy diet, your targeted supplement regimen, and your rest and relaxation prescription. You are ready to begin—and we couldn't be more thrilled for you.

Many of our patients find that the first 6 weeks of the program can be tricky—as we all know, change can be really tough! So to get you over the 6-week hurdle, we've created a set of week-by-week strategies, each one packed with specific tips for that particular stage of those critical first weeks. Read through the next chapter for a heads-up on what's coming your way.

THE FIRST 6 WEEKS

Successful weight loss requires more than eating differently, resting, and taking supplements. To drop pounds and keep them off, you must embrace change—lots of change. And as you know if you've tried to lose weight before, change isn't easy. In fact, it's stressful. It requires letting go of your past comforts and habits and embracing new habits and strategies.

To help you form new habits and stick with them, we've created this guide for your first 6 weeks and beyond. It walks you through the tough times, helping you find the motivation you need to stick with change when all you want to do is return to your old, familiar weight-gaining ways.

Are you ready to work hard? Then get ready to lose big.

DAY 1

Start the plan on a low-key day. Consider starting it on a weekend, if your weekends are less stressful than your weekdays. Definitely start it the day after a grocery run, so that all of your supplies are on hand. Follow these tips for your three main meals.

Breakfast: Unless otherwise noted in Chapter 9, take your supplements after breakfast. This is the easiest time to remember them. If you are not in the habit of eating breakfast, grab a mozzarella cheese stick, some celery or cucumbers, or a couple of hard-boiled eggs. Remember: Breakfast is the most important meal to do right. Don't skip it, and don't set yourself up for an incredibly hard day by having a doughnut or Danish.

Midday: If you're the type of person who gets absorbed in work and forgets to eat lunch, set an alarm on your watch, cell phone, or computer to remind you to stop and eat. Ignore the intruding thought that will no doubt whisper, "I don't have time to eat lunch." Replace it with the thought, "I don't have time *not* to eat lunch." Also, remind yourself that you will make up for the time you took to eat by being more productive in the afternoon. Most people work more effectively after they've eaten.

Dinner: Because you fueled yourself throughout the day with healthful fats, protein, and fiber, you'll be less likely than usual to over-eat at dinner and afterward. That's a plus. On the minus side, however, dinner usually presents unique challenges for most people. First, you have the temptation of seeing your dining companions' plates filled with foods that you may be trying to avoid. If you come home from work or other daytime activities feeling tired, you have the temptation of ordering in food that may not conform to this diet.

To reduce temptations, plan your dinner menu ahead of time. Have quick and easy options on hand. Most important, eat dinner mindfully.

Eat more frequently if you notice hunger and cravings. Don't try to ride these out. Keep convenient options on hand, such as precooked meatballs, roasted turkey, hard-boiled eggs, and so on. When you feel hungry, eat. These between-meal hunger pangs and cravings will probably subside within 4 days, once your body switches into fat-burning mode.

DAYS 2 THROUGH 6

Some people coast through the first week of the diet without any problems. With each progressive day, they feel better and better as they fuel their bodies with real food and stop sending their insulin and blood sugar on roller-coaster rides. Others encounter mild to severe withdrawal symptoms. These may be a necessary evil, but they are not everlasting. You may be recovering from two addictions during the first week.

1. **Carbohydrate addiction: If you've been surviving on a very low-fat, very high-carbohydrate diet that's loaded with sugar,**

high-fructose corn syrup, and refined flour, your body has gotten used to the peaks and valleys this diet has inflicted on your blood sugar levels. For you, high insulin and high blood sugar may feel normal, even though both are neither normal nor good. As you get used to the sensation of normal levels of blood sugar and insulin, you may initially feel tired, get headaches, and be irritable.

2. **Caffeine addiction: If you are weaning yourself off a high-caffeine lifestyle, then you may notice withdrawal symptoms during the first week of this major change.** Take acetaminophen for headaches and try L-glutamine (500 milligrams before meals up to three times a day) or a B complex supplement (100 milligrams once a day) to reduce cravings for caffeine.

Even if you are not addicted to carbs or caffeine, you may still notice some unpleasant symptoms during week 1 as your body switches from burning carbohydrates to burning fat for fuel. Before it switches to fat burning, your body will first burn through the stores of carbohydrates in your muscles and liver. The length of time it takes to exhaust these stores varies from person to person. If you are very active, your body may switch to fat burning as quickly as within the first 24 hours on the diet. If you are very sedentary, it might take as long as 3 or 4 days. As your metabolism is getting used to this new fuel source, you may experience some fatigue and headaches. Once you switch completely to a fat-burning metabolism, however, you can expect to feel a lot more energy. This is why we recommend you start the diet during a low-key week.

It's extremely important to stick to your guns and follow the diet precisely during week 1. This will help your body adjust to burning fat as fuel. If you continually sneak in a few extra carbs each day, you'll prolong negative side effects, and your weight loss may even stall. Once your body burns through its stores of carbohydrates, you can more easily stray from the plan without suffering any ill effects. You basically have more room to cheat.

Here are the best remedies for the initial withdrawal symptoms.

■ **Patience.** It's just a few days. Mark them off on the calendar with huge Xs.

- **Naps.** Take mini rests during the day as needed. Ten minutes of relaxation or a short nap can do wonders.
- **Eating.** Have a high-fat, high-protein, or high-fiber snack whenever you feel tired, hungry, or irritable. Try a scoop of chicken salad and a few slices of avocado, a cheese stick wrapped in turkey, sliced olives in egg salad, or celery with peanut butter.

DAY 7

Congratulations on completing your first week on the diet! If you have not already stepped onto the scale, we have some advice for you. Hold off until after you read this! You probably have a number in your head that you'd like to see on the scale. Maybe you were hoping to lose 2 pounds. Perhaps 5. Maybe it's 10. Try to put that number completely out of your mind. We'd love to tell you what number to expect today, but we just can't. Everyone loses weight at a different pace. The speed with which the pounds drop off depends on a number of factors, including:

Your starting weight. The heavier you are, the faster your metabolism, and the more dramatic your initial weight loss. In other words, you lose more because you have more to lose.

Your health. A metabolic disadvantage such as an insulin disadvantage will slow weight loss, particularly in the beginning. All of the disadvantages slow weight loss, but the insulin and thyroid disadvantages probably slow it the most.

Your age and gender. Postmenopausal women tend to lose weight more slowly than younger women or men of any age.

Your former eating habits. If you lived on cheese doodles, potato chips, and Twinkies, you'll probably lose more initial weight than someone who was already eating whole foods.

The point is this: If you followed the plan during week 1, it doesn't matter what number you see on the scale. Congratulate yourself for getting through a very hard week. You are now 7 days closer to forming new, permanent eating habits. You've gotten through the hardest of times—you've survived the withdrawal symptoms. If you already feel more energy, that's great. If not, you can expect to feel more and more energetic with each passing day. Your mood should improve as well. Of course, the number on the scale is important, but so is the way you feel.

Now that you've read that pep talk, go to it. Go to the bathroom and step on the scale. Celebrate that weight loss, and commit yourself to another week of losing.

DAYS 8 THROUGH 13

Your week 2 strategy is the same as that for week 1: Stick to the plan! As one of our clients has said, you must approach weight loss as you approach investments: Buy into a plan and hold for the long term.

Expect week 2 to feel slightly easier than week 1. You're somewhat used to your eating choices now, so it may take less effort to prepare your meals. Any side effects you experienced during week 1 should have subsided. If you have a metabolic disadvantage such as an insulin disadvantage, you should be feeling better than you have in months or years. Use that extra energy and improved mood as motivation to stay the course.

If you deviate from the food options, recommit to the plan right away. Don't wait until the next day—or worse, the following week—to resume weight loss. The faster you recommit, the more weight you'll continue to lose. And, no matter how long you go off the wagon, don't give up. Just get back on.

Also, now is not the time to get cocky. We know people who lost 7 or 10 pounds during week 1 and thought, "I just lost 7 pounds. This is easy. I can ease up. I can deviate from the plan and still lose." In a word: no. You lose a lot of weight at first on this plan because you lose water along with fat. Your weight loss will slow slightly over the next few weeks. You might have lost up to 10 pounds during week 1, but in the next few weeks your weight loss will be slower. You must follow the plan to continually see rewards on the scale.

DAY 14

Congratulations on your 2-week weight-loss anniversary. You're doing great. Go ahead and step on the scale. Do a little victory dance, and then come back to the book. We'll wait.

Now that you are 2 weeks into the plan, it's time to reassess the situation. Can you keep this up? How do you feel about your food choices? If you feel good about the way you are eating, stick with it. If, on the other hand, you are dreaming about something sweet after dinner or toast in the morning or an occasional glass of wine, let's talk about it. If you are feeling deprived now, just 2 weeks into the plan, you can only expect that feeling of deprivation to strengthen. You might make it a few more weeks without indulging, but, eventually, your willpower will erode. That's why you really have to use your daily indulgences. Have you been eating them? If not, definitely start. If so, maybe you should consider moving up to Level 2, to broaden your horizons with luxury foods. If you try to ignore your cravings, they'll intensify. You'll eat more, you'll feel worse about yourself, and you'll have a harder time maintaining your momentum.

Think about what it is about high–carbohydrate foods that you really miss. Is it the crunch? Do you miss bread more than anything? Or do you just need something sweet every once in a while? Think about it and be honest. It's different for everyone. Once you come up with your answer, read on.

If you need something sweet: Use the fruit or chocolate option we provide, even in Level 1. Save your fruit for the time of day you most like to have something sweet. For many people, that's right after dinner. Indulge in your sweet treat when you are relatively full. This will prevent you from overdoing it. In lieu of fruit, try mixing various types of spices into ricotta cheese. We prefer cinnamon because it tends to improve blood sugar, but cardamom, cocoa, vanilla, mint, and other sweet spices and herbs can work just as well. You can also drizzle up to 1 tablespoon of sugar-free chocolate syrup on top.

If you need more crunch: Have one low-carb, thin crisp cracker (such Wasa or Kavli) as a snack when you need the crunch. Smear it with guacamole, apple butter, peanut butter, or some other low-carb spread. Other good options include raw vegetables, celery with cream cheese or blue cheese dressing, sliced cucumber, and Baked Cheese (page 235).

If you need something savory: Allow yourself the slice of bread for Level 1! Don't take low-carb eating to extremes. We've done the math for you. You can have bread and still induce fat burning. We know it's hard to believe, but it's true. Either toast and butter it or smear it with guacamole, apple butter, or trans fats–free peanut butter. Also, plan a special meal, such as lobster with asparagus or filet mignon with steamed broccoli.

If you need more satisfaction: Are you allowing yourself to eat fat? We ask because many of our clients struggle with this plan when they try to simultaneously make it low carb and low fat. But as Harvard's Walter Willett, PhD, has said time and time again, it's the types of fat (nonhydrogenated) and the types of carbs (nonprocessed whole foods) that matter to good health. Fat is healthy. All of our patients got healthier on this plan.

Allow yourself to indulge in fat. If you love guacamole, have it. If it's butter that satisfies you, have it. If it's cream, have it. You need to satisfy that part of yourself that loves food. Don't deprive yourself of fat. There's no need to be miserable. Yes, you have to cut back on some foods—such as processed fats, hydrogenated fats, and more—but don't cut back on even more than we require on this plan. It's not worth it, and it's not necessary.

If you have a metabolic disadvantage—particularly an insulin disadvantage—we recommend you follow Level 1 for at least a month. That's the length of time you need to improve your metabolism. If, however, following the plan for an entire month means you risk relapsing and quitting the plan altogether, then consider moving up to Level 2 for a week or two, and then back down to Level 1. Many of our patients lost all of their weight this way, switching between the different level plans as life unfolded around them. Make it work for you. Stick with the plan that accommodates your metabolic type most of the time, but move up to more liberal plans as needed. Although your success hinges on consistency, it ultimately involves finding out what works for you.

WEEK 2

Have you heard that you should chew gum or refocus your thoughts to avoid giving in to a craving? Do you want to know what we think of that advice? Hogwash. If you are hungry or craving food, eat. Just eat according to plan. Stay full. That's the best way to keep yourself away from the bagels, scones, and other foods that tend to unravel your sense of control. If you are hungry or having a craving, eat a small meal such as a few meatballs, a hard-boiled egg, some turkey wrapped with cheese, or vegetables with cream cheese. If you tend to get cravings at the same time of day, eat one of these snacks 30 minutes before you typically notice the craving.

WEEK 3

It may not happen this week, but it will happen: Your new eating habits will collide with your social life, family life, or career. At some point, you will go out to eat with your spouse or friends and just have to have a taste of dessert or a glass of wine. At some point, you will encounter a holiday table covered with bread, stuffing, apple crisp, and other foods you don't find listed on the Level 1 or 2 plans. At some point, you'll go on vacation or travel for business and have few food options.

What to do? You do the best you can. Here are some strategies.

Move up to Level 2. We created two levels, in part, so you could have some flexibility. When you know you'll be traveling, at a holiday party, or somewhere that you cannot follow the diet to a T, plan for indulgence. If you are following Level 1, move up to Level 2. If you're already on Level 2, pick a plan that might fit the menu that evening. If you've already transitioned up from Level 2, allow yourself one extra serving of a carbohydrate food you love. Don't expect the pounds to melt away as you follow a less-restrictive plan, but do expect to maintain or even lose a little.

Follow the indulgence food plan guidelines. A glass of wine with dinner once a week probably won't halt your weight loss. Occasionally splitting a small dessert with a friend or loved one probably won't either. When our patients follow the plans, we're delighted! We tell them, "Good for you!" You need to indulge from time to time. That's life. That's love. That's happiness.

The danger here is when an occasional indulgence, even a planned one, turns into a daily indulgence: One small indulgence (a glass of wine) turns into an entire meal or day of excess. If you are having a special meal, choose one indulgence for the day and then follow that plan. It might be a glass of wine. It might be having a roll from the bread basket (with butter or dipped in oil, please!) with the rest of your dining companions. It might be a small, starchy carbohydrate side dish such as a baked potato. It might be splitting a dessert with your dining companion. It's just not doing *all* of that.

Don't be afraid to throw food away. Nearly all of our patients have learned to stay in control by eating tempting foods away from home. They order one small serving, savor it, and walk away. If you do, however, have something tempting in your home—perhaps because a friend or family member put it there—don't be afraid to use your trash can to help you stay in control. "If you eat a slice of pie or cake or something else and there's a huge amount left over, throw the rest away," recommends Dave, one of our patients. "You'll be much less likely to pick it out of the garbage so you can have another slice, and usually, once it's out of sight, it's out of mind. If you put it in the fridge, you'll end up having another slice the next day. If you feel guilty when throwing away food, think of it this way: You probably throw away fruits and vegetables all the time. Why are cake, cookies, and other desserts any different?"

Keep tabs on how you feel, particularly the day after an indulgence. This will go a long way toward making your new eating plan a permanent habit. If you indulged a little too much at dinner last night—say, in addition to the wine, you also had a cannoli and you split it with no one—you'll probably wake the next day feeling less than your usual self. You might have a headache. You might feel lethargic. You may even feel as if you are getting a cold or the flu. Take notice. This is your body's way of telling you that you overdid it. You probably felt this way all the time before starting this diet. It was such a consistent sensation that you did not realize how food was affecting you. By now, 3 weeks into the plan, you should be feeling pretty good. When you overdo it, your body will tell you. If you listen, you'll be less likely to overdo it in the future because, in addition to knowing how those foods affect your waistline, you'll know how they affect your energy levels and overall sense of well-being.

Get right back on track, with the strictest plan. If, despite your best efforts, you completely go overboard—having pasta, alcohol, and dessert—get back on track as soon as possible. Stop the mind-set that says, "I cheated, I might as well keep on cheating." Replace it with the mind-set that says, "Okay, so I overdid it. Now I'll make up for it by sticking to the plan better than before." If you've been following Level 2, drop down to Level 1 for a day or two to make up for the overindulgence. Even with Level 1, omit the fruit, oatmeal, or bread options. For 1 or 2 days, consume only meat, eggs, fish, and vegetables. This not only will keep weight loss going, but it also will help you deal with any guilty feelings that may tempt you to stop dieting altogether.

Know yourself. We all have trigger foods that are addictive. Not only can you not hold yourself to a reasonable portion of these foods, but they also actually induce physical sensations, such as sweating and a racing heartbeat. If you want to indulge in chocolate but you know you cannot stop at two squares, then do not indulge in chocolate. If you have an insulin disadvantage, this is extremely important because any dessert has the potential to swing your blood sugar up and down, triggering intense cravings for more sweets.

Make the best choice you can in any given situation, get back on the plan as soon as possible, and look at ways to solve the problem that caused you to go off the plan in the first place. If you start to plateau at this point, skip ahead to Week 6.

WEEK 4

Remember how motivated you were on day 1? You're almost a month into the plan now. You may have lost 10 or more pounds. You're probably feeling fantastic. Friends may be commenting on changes they see in your body.

To keep your motivation going, now is a good time to take stock of all of the positive changes these new eating habits have brought you. Take a moment to think about how you've changed in the following areas:

- Sleep habits: Do you fall asleep more easily and sleep more deeply?
- Stress: Do you feel more relaxed and calm?
- Mood: Do you feel happier and more even-tempered?
- Energy: Do you feel less sleepy in the afternoon? Do you feel as if you can accomplish more in a given day?
- Confidence: Do you feel as if you can do anything? (*We* know you can. Do *you* know it?)

Now is also a good time to think about why you are trying to lose weight. Four weeks ago, you had your reasons. Maybe you wanted to look good for a special occasion. Maybe you wanted to do it because your doctor put the fear of God into you. Maybe you wanted to do it for your spouse or a loved one.

To keep up the momentum long term, however, you need to do this for yourself. If you started this journey for someone else, you will eventually hit a wall. The effort required to lose weight will eventually override your desire to please this person, and you'll at some point decide that weight loss just is not worth the effort. On the other hand, if you are doing this for you, you *are* worth the effort—always. It has to be for you and not for your boyfriend and not to win the approval of your wife.

So why are you doing this? Why is weight loss important to you? For many people, it has to do with three benefits: improved health, improved well-being, and improved self-confidence. Really, losing weight is similar to any huge effort. It's tough work. If you lose weight and keep it off, you should feel as proud of yourself as if you ran a marathon, wrote a symphony, wrote a book, or earned a higher education degree. It requires persistence, dedication, and endurance. You are worth it. Do it because you believe in yourself and want better for yourself.

WEEK 5

We'd like you to consider a very important question: Are you doing this alone? If you are, realize that your journey will be more difficult than if you had more support. Research shows that solo dieters tend to have higher levels of the stress hormone cortisol than dieters who have more support.

Support starts with family, but it also encompasses friends and coworkers. Support comes from people who want you to reach your dreams. In this case, the dream is a smaller clothing size. In the future, the dream may be a career change, a pregnancy, or a financial goal. It really doesn't matter what the dream is, because all dreams require effort. All dreams require change. All dreams require you to reach deep down into yourself and turn yourself into a different, stronger, better person.

Some people in your life will cheer you on as you go through this metamorphosis. Others will feel threatened, and they will cling to the old you. They may express their loss in subtle ways, perhaps through comments about meals they'd like to eat with you. Some express it in outright sabotage, buying cookies and other treats and presenting them to you to eat.

Weight loss is hard, and few people can do it alone. It's even harder if you have people in your life who actively work against your efforts. To determine your level of support, answer yes or no to each of the following questions.

1. Is your spouse or significant other overweight?

☐ YES   ☐ NO

2. Is food the center of family gatherings, celebrations, or events?

☐ YES   ☐ NO

3. Has your spouse or significant other sabotaged your efforts to lose weight in the past (for example, by stocking the freezer with ice cream or by asking you to have a cookie)?

☐ YES   ☐ NO

4. Do family members put you in situations that may increase your likelihood of falling off your nutrition plan?

☐ YES   ☐ NO

5. Is your spouse jealous of your weight loss?

☐ YES   ☐ NO

6. Are most of your friends overweight?

☐ YES   ☐ NO

7. Do you usually catch up with friends over dinner, a drink, or dessert?

☐ YES   ☐ NO

8. Are your friends jealous of your weight loss?

☐ YES   ☐ NO

9. Do your friends sometimes bake you sweets as gifts?

☐ YES   ☐ NO

10. Do coworkers keep tempting foods in plain sight?

☐ YES   ☐ NO

11. Do coworkers give you sweets and other tempting foods as gifts?

☐ YES   ☐ NO

12. Do coworkers leave food in a break room for others to share?

☐ YES   ☐ NO

13. Are most of your coworkers overweight?

☐ YES   ☐ NO

If you answered yes to any of those questions, you could stand to line up more support for yourself. Here are some strategies for garnering more support.

Ask for it. Explain why you want to lose weight. Explain why weight loss is important for you, and ask family, friends, and coworkers to support your efforts.

Share your diet with your family. If you eat one way while everyone else in the family eats another way, you won't stay on the diet for long. There's no reason not to introduce this way of eating to your entire family. We're talking about real food. More than one in five kids is overweight, and type 2 diabetes affects kids as young as age 4. Both overweight and diabetes are related to diets rich in processed foods and fast food. To get your kids on board, introduce pure foods such as fresh fruit, vegetables, and other whole foods. The only reason children like Twinkies is because grown-ups let them taste them. We know kids who say, "McDonald's? That's yucky!" That's because their parents taught them this view, and, more important, never took them to a fast food restaurant during their formative years. Get your kids involved in choosing healthful foods when shopping. Let them put the carrots, apples, and other foods in the cart. Save less-healthy snacks for special occasions.

If you have small children, start a "sometimes" rule. We learned this trick from Dave, a patient who lost 40 pounds. "I noticed that my kids were eating fries and sugary cereals and ice cream three times a day. My wife and I decided that these foods could be sometimes foods, but they weren't going to be everyday treats. The kids could have them every once in a while, but their three main meals were going to consist of real, whole foods. They still ask for the ice cream, of course, but I don't feel guilty because they've slimmed down since we started the sometimes rule. It's had a positive effect on the whole family."

Find a weight-loss buddy. Runners often train for marathons with a partner or group. College students form study groups. People who are climbing the corporate ladder usually have one or two coworkers who share their frustrations and accomplishments. Why do so many people try to lose weight in secret? We recommend you find a weight-loss buddy. If your spouse or a close friend or family member is overweight, this may be as simple as embarking on the plan together. Also consider going to a weight-related support group or finding a buddy online.

In addition to lining up more support, you also must learn how to deal with difficult people. Otherwise, naysayers can easily erode your willpower.

Below, we've listed some common obstacles and how to overcome them.

Someone offers you food that you are trying not to eat. Saying no requires you to put aside your need to please others. Be assertive. Say something like, "I feel flattered that you thought to bring me this food. I am trying hard to lose weight, however, and this food is not one I can eat. I feel horrible that I need to turn away your offer, but I hope you understand." If this person is a true friend or supporter, he or she will sympathize. Friends and loved ones should want to help us grow into our better selves. If you feel guilty about turning down these requests to eat, realize that the friend or loved one is the person who should feel guilty: That person is the one who is blocking you from growing into a better you.

Your spouse or children complain about the new and different foods you put on the dinner table. They may also gripe about your not wanting to go out to eat as much as you used to. Whatever the situation, you must be firm and assertive. Explain why weight loss is important to you. Ask your family to help you come up with a common solution. Perhaps they could pitch in and help cook certain foods. Perhaps you can find nonfood-focused ways to enjoy time together, such as watching a sporting event or going for a walk after dinner. If you focus on finding solutions to these issues, you'll be able to work through them.

Your spouse complains that he or she misses the old you. Invite your spouse to get to know the new you. Take time to really hear about each other's dreams, opinions, and values. Perhaps your spouse does not have the dream of weight loss, but he or she has some kind of dream. Everyone has a dream. If you can find this common ground, you can support one another.

You feel out of touch with your spouse. Many married couples know one another through food. Perhaps you used to share a doughnut run one weekend morning or an ice cream run on a particular night. When you go on a diet, these shared activities may stop, but that doesn't mean you can't spend time together! Many clients worry that they don't know how to relate to one another if food is not the center of the relationship. You know what she suggests? What better way to reconnect with one another than in the bedroom? Valerie, for example, counseled one couple who used to bond with an ice cream run. When they gave it up they felt as if something was missing in their relationship. When they swapped the run for sex, they grew closer and were much happier. If you really want to have fun, get sugar-free chocolate syrup, on each other!

for long. There's no reason not to introduce this way of eating to your entire family. We're talking about real food. More than one in five kids is overweight, and type 2 diabetes affects kids as young as age 4. Both overweight and diabetes are related to diets rich in processed foods and fast food. To get your kids on board, introduce pure foods such as fresh fruit, vegetables, and other whole foods. The only reason children like Twinkies is because grown-ups let them taste them. We know kids who say, "McDonald's? That's yucky!" That's because their parents taught them this view, and, more important, never took them to a fast food restaurant during their formative years. Get your kids involved in choosing healthful foods when shopping. Let them put the carrots, apples, and other foods in the cart. Save less-healthy snacks for special occasions.

If you have small children, start a "sometimes" rule. We learned this trick from Dave, a patient who lost 40 pounds. "I noticed that my kids were eating fries and sugary cereals and ice cream three times a day. My wife and I decided that these foods could be sometimes foods, but they weren't going to be everyday treats. The kids could have them every once in a while, but their three main meals were going to consist of real, whole foods. They still ask for the ice cream, of course, but I don't feel guilty because they've slimmed down since we started the sometimes rule. It's had a positive effect on the whole family."

Find a weight-loss buddy. Runners often train for marathons with a partner or group. College students form study groups. People who are climbing the corporate ladder usually have one or two coworkers who share their frustrations and accomplishments. Why do so many people try to lose weight in secret? We recommend you find a weight-loss buddy. If your spouse or a close friend or family member is overweight, this may be as simple as embarking on the plan together. Also consider going to a weight-related support group or finding a buddy online.

In addition to lining up more support, you also must learn how to deal with difficult people. Otherwise, naysayers can easily erode your willpower.

Below, we've listed some common obstacles and how to overcome them.

Someone offers you food that you are trying not to eat. Saying no requires you to put aside your need to please others. Be assertive. Say something like, "I feel flattered that you thought to bring me this food. I am trying hard to lose weight, however, and this food is not one I can eat. I feel horrible that I need to turn away your offer, but I hope you understand." If this person is a true friend or supporter, he or she will sympathize. Friends and loved ones should want to help us grow into our better selves. If you feel guilty about turning down these requests to eat, realize that the friend or loved one is the person who should feel guilty: That person is the one who is blocking you from growing into a better you.

Your spouse or children complain about the new and different foods you put on the dinner table. They may also gripe about your not wanting to go out to eat as much as you used to. Whatever the situation, you must be firm and assertive. Explain why weight loss is important to you. Ask your family to help you come up with a common solution. Perhaps they could pitch in and help cook certain foods. Perhaps you can find nonfood-focused ways to enjoy time together, such as watching a sporting event or going for a walk after dinner. If you focus on finding solutions to these issues, you'll be able to work through them.

Your spouse complains that he or she misses the old you. Invite your spouse to get to know the new you. Take time to really hear about each other's dreams, opinions, and values. Perhaps your spouse does not have the dream of weight loss, but he or she has some kind of dream. Everyone has a dream. If you can find this common ground, you can support one another.

You feel out of touch with your spouse. Many married couples know one another through food. Perhaps you used to share a doughnut run one weekend morning or an ice cream run on a particular night. When you go on a diet, these shared activities may stop, but that doesn't mean you can't spend time together! Many clients tell Valerie that they don't know how to relate to one another if food is not at the center of the relationship. You know what she suggests? Sex. What better way to reconnect with one another than in the bedroom? Valerie, for example, counseled one couple who used to bond at 2 a.m. with an ice cream run. When they gave it up, they felt as if something was missing in their relationship. When they swapped the ice cream run for sex, they grew closer and were much happier for it. If you really want to have fun, get sugar-free chocolate syrup and drizzle it on each other!

Here are some other ways to reconnect:

- See a movie together.
- Go for a long drive through the country.
- Play a board game or do a crossword puzzle together.
- Attend a cultural event.

We suspect you'll eventually find that these nonfood activities are a lot more fun and enriching than those ice cream runs!

Your spouse feels jealous of your better-looking body. Your spouse may worry that if you look more attractive, you'll attract potential suitors. Assuage this fear by reminding your spouse why you love him or her. What do you find attractive about his or her personality, values, and opinions?

Your spouse doesn't know how to please you without food. Some romantic partners will bring you food as gifts. Explain that you would prefer something other than food. Make a list of nonfood gifts you would like to receive, such as flowers, a massage, lingerie, and so on.

Your spouse sabotages you. I've had clients whose spouses have not only resisted getting certain trigger foods out of the house, but have also gone as far as to ask the dieter to buy these foods at the store! If this is the case, explain that these foods are like an addiction for you and that you are trying to lose weight for your health. Your spouse may not really want you to succeed, and you need to talk about why.

WEEK 6

Whether it happens this week or at some other point, there will come a time when you get on the scale and find that you've lost very little or no weight at all. You may have lost a lot in the beginning. Perhaps you lost 10 pounds the first week, another 10 the next, and then 2 or so each week after that. At some point, 2 will turn to 1 and then to zero.

Plateaus are common and everyone reaches one eventually. When you reach a plateau, try not to be distressed. We know this is hard, but as long as you are sticking to your plan, then you will eventually start losing again. We've seen this happen time and time again. For example, Valerie recently worked with a client named Guy. He had lost 20 pounds, but then plateaued roughly 15 pounds short of his goal. He stuck to his guns and continued to follow the diet. Guy had kept a

Guy Lost **40 Pounds!**

When I came to Valerie, I was exercising as much as an hour a day—but I couldn't lose weight. It was frustrating, to say the least.

After meeting with Valerie, I realized that some of my eating habits were interfering with my efforts to lose weight. My eating, for one, was hit or miss. I was and still am a very busy businessman. I often skipped meals. I just forgot to eat.

Then I'd eat dinner at a restaurant and would make up for it—and then some.

It took a few key changes in my eating habits for my weight to start coming off. I began eating regular meals, eating more vegetables, and eating less starch and sugar. I never felt deprived. I even had the occasional glass of wine, and I continued to lose.

After I lost 20 pounds, though, I plateaued. I was 15 pounds short of my goal.

I knew I could change things up. I could get stricter with my eating or try to exercise even more, but I went with a concept I'd learned in business. I decided to buy and hold long term. It worked.

Two months later, I started losing again and eventually I hit my goal weight. I'm healthier and fitter than I've ever been, too.

detailed food log since day 1 of the diet, so we looked over the log. He was doing everything right, and he felt good about how he was eating. We could have made his eating plan stricter, but we decided to wait and see. Two months later, he started losing again.

Start keeping a food diary and be honest with yourself. You may feel tempted to not write down certain foods you wish you had not eaten. Anytime you feel the urge to not write something down, that's exactly when you *should* be writing it down. Look over your log each day for hidden saboteurs. Common ones include:

- Commercially prepared meatballs and tuna salad that might contain excess soy fillers
- Commercial salad dressings that contain high-fructose corn syrup and partially hydrogenated fats
- Commercially prepared yogurt that contains cane sugar or high-fructose corn syrup
- Commercially prepared coleslaw that contains added sugar
- Imitation crabmeat that contains added sugar
- Deli meats that have extra nitrates or glutamates
- Packets of artificial sweeteners that may have amped up your sweet tooth

If you have a yeast disadvantage, pay attention to yeast-forming foods that may have crept back into your diet. Are you consuming balsamic vinegar again? Have you started drinking coffee again? Sun-dried tomatoes also tend to exacerbate yeast problems in some people, possibly because of the processing or added nitrates.

Also, be careful with the serving sizes of cheese and nuts—remember that these foods do have carbs. Many people tend to overdo these foods, especially cheese.

If, after examining your records, you see you are doing everything right, you have two options.

Option 1: Just hold on. Some experts believe that plateaus happen because the metabolism slows as your body grows smaller. If this were the case, however, the plateau would be your final resting point. We've counseled hundreds of dieters who did nothing to change what they were eating and eventually started losing again. So something else is going on. You may be losing, just more slowly. Perhaps you're losing ¼ pound each week. This small loss won't show up until 4 weeks later, after each ¼ pound has added up to a pound. Also, if you are exercising, you may be swapping fat for muscle—muscle is more compact but weighs more than fat. Guy, for example, noticed that his clothes continued to get baggier, even though his weight wasn't changing on the scale.

Option 2: Get stricter. If you need the motivation of a dropping number or shrinking body, then step down a level. If you are at Level 2, go to Level 1. If you are at Level 1, cut back on one of the carbohydrate servings, such as the ½ cup of fruit. Unless you have a thyroid or an adrenal disadvantage, try logging your food intake to make sure you are eating what you think you are eating. Also, get a checkup to see whether some other medical problem is blocking further weight loss.

UNTIL YOU REACH YOUR GOAL

Now you know almost everything you need to know to lose all of the weight you want. We'll leave you with some parting advice.

- Whenever you struggle, come back to the book. All the evidence you need that what you're doing is worth it is right here. Reread some of the earlier chapters that explain the reasons why you're not only losing weight but also saving your life. Talk about motivation!

- If you feel deprived or you dream about going off the plan, it's time to make a modification. Try another indulgence food. Reread the advice for weeks 2 and 3, and experiment with adding in extra or different foods. What can you add to the plan to make it work for you?
- As you near your weight loss goal, allow more variety into your eating repertoire. Add one new food or an extra serving of a specific food once every 2 weeks, and notice how you feel as you add foods back in. Start with whole foods such as beans, lentils, fruit, starchy vegetables (such as sweet potatoes), nuts and seeds, and so on. If you've been holding out on trying an indulgence food, now's the time. Keep tabs on your weight and how you feel. You must carefully balance indulgence with what your body can handle. Some people can indulge more than others and continue to lose weight. Others cannot. You'll find more advice for reintroducing foods in Chapter 13.

WHEN AND HOW
TO BE ACTIVE

Many of our patients are ecstatic when we suggest they not attempt to exercise until after they've lost some weight. Although exercise is important for many, many reasons—and we'll go into some of them in this chapter—it does not have to be your first weight loss priority, especially if you are the type of person who has hated exercise since your very first elementary school gym class.

Here's why. First, you already have a lot on your mind. You are changing your eating habits, for one. You're taking new supplements, and you are incorporating new stress-reduction tactics. This all requires a large amount of mental energy. Change of any kind is hard. Change, in fact, is stressful. Trying to change your eating habits and start an exercise program simultaneously is a recipe for one thing—more mental stress. We want you to feel less stress, not more.

Second, if you are more than 20 pounds above your ideal body weight, exercise may even cause you pain. Those extra pounds put a great deal of pressure on your joints. Starting a program now may even lead to injury.

Finally, if you have any of the metabolic disadvantages described in Chapter 5, you probably don't have the energy to start an exercise program. Ideally, exercise should make you feel better, not worse. If you feel exhausted after exercise, you do not yet have the physical reserves needed to complete an exercise session. For you, exercise is the equivalent of trying to drive across the country on an empty gas tank. Let's fill your tank by fixing the underlying metabolic problems with diet, supplements, and rest. Once you fill your tank, you'll have the energy you need to get moving.

WHY EXERCISE HELPS

Most studies show that dietary changes result in up to three times the amount of weight loss as increasing your exercise time does. Think of food as your bridge to a leaner, healthier body. Without that bridge, you can't get from point A (an unhealthy, overweight body) to point B (a healthy, lean body).

Think of movement as the railings that allow you to stay on your food bridge. These railings help ensure that you stay firmly planted on the point B side of the bridge once you get across. Exercise keeps you on the bridge by helping you:

Preserve muscle mass. Some of the weight you lose during any weight loss program will come from muscle, slowing your metabolism. Exercise, particularly weight training, helps preserve muscle mass so your metabolism stays strong as you lose weight. This helps prevent weight regain once you reach your goal.

Make weight loss stick. Results from the National Weight

Morris "Moshe" Jacobs **Lost 30 Pounds!**

When I turned 60, I found myself overweight, out of shape, and in poor health. I wanted to start a new life and get back into shape. The motivation I needed came one day when I visited my general practitioner. He told me that I had high blood pressure and was developing diabetes. He gave me an ultimatum. He told me I had one month to lose weight or he would put me on more medication.

I'd lost weight before on many different crazy diets, but I'd always put it back on. I knew Keith through a business relationship. I needed something that would stick. I walked out of my GP's office, got in my car, and drove straight to Keith's office. The first thing he told me was, "Don't worry. We'll fix you up. Everything is manageable. Don't be frightened."

He suggested an eating approach, along with some supplements. I now eat very little sugar and flour. I have multigrain crackers every once in a while, or wild rice, but I limit the quantities. When I'm hungry I have almonds or avocado. That keeps me feeling full. Once in a blue moon I'll have some ice cream. I

Q: *Doesn't exercise incinerate calories?*

A: You must run or walk an entire mile to burn just 100 calories. One pound of fat contains 3,500 calories. So, to burn a pound of fat each week, you'd have to run the equivalent of 5 miles every day. Compare that to dietary changes, which net you anywhere between a 2- and a 10-pound drop in weight week after week after week.

Control Registry—a long-term study of thousands of people who have lost more than 30 pounds and kept it off for a year or longer—show that nearly all of the successful losers exercised to keep off the weight.

Boost mood. Exercise raises levels of brain chemicals that elevate mood. This makes you more likely to stick with your eating habits, because the happier you are, the less emotional eating you will do.

Stay healthy. Exercise helps sensitize the body to many different hormones, including insulin and cortisol. This ensures that, once you mend your metabolism, the right amount and right types of exercise will keep you healthy.

Reduce stress. A Hungarian study of 207 men and women shows

crave it a lot less now. I don't miss it. Once in a while I have it, but it doesn't destroy me on the days I go without it, either.

It wasn't hard for me because I was so determined to get well. I think of it as a former smoker or a former drinker might think of his or her vices. I'm so happy to be healthy, but there's probably a part of me that will always yearn for the foods I limit. Because I'm doing this for my health, I find it easier to stay in control. I feel so good now. I don't want to get sick again.

I lost a significant amount of weight and my sugar levels came down, too. This plan got me off one blood pressure medication and is helping me reduce the dosage of a second.

I now weigh 153 pounds. I have so much energy. I exercise four times a week, and I've never felt better in my life. I love it. I always wanted to exercise before, but this is the first time I've had the energy to sustain a structured program. I feel so much better. I'm no longer exhausted.

Now I can keep up with my grandkids. When they want to play ball, I'm there with them.

that people who are physically fit tend to have fewer inflammatory responses to mental stressors than people who are out of shape.

Stay young. Exercise improves heart health. A stronger heart can more effectively pump blood—and oxygen—to all parts of your body.

HOW TO EXERCISE

If you are already fit, you may be able to continue the exercise you're doing or slightly modify what you're doing and still lose weight. We're in no way telling you to stop exercising. Rather, we're telling you that starting an exercise program should not be your first priority.

If you are currently sedentary, we've outlined an exercise program in the following pages that will take you from beginner to advanced. You'll progress in three steps: You'll start by building flexibility and balance, progress to building strength, and finish by adding cardiovascular conditioning. This is the specific exercise routine that we recommend to our patients. Start this program only after you feel in control of your new dietary habits.

Program 1

Best For:

- Anyone with an adrenal disadvantage
- Anyone with more than 20 pounds to lose
- Anyone who is currently out of shape

Start Program 1 only when you feel ready. Focus first on changing your eating, de-stressing, and taking your supplements. Once those changes no longer feel overwhelming, then you are ready for movement. In Program 1, we'd like you to incorporate two kinds of activity into your life.

Mental activity. If you don't already take part in a hobby, think about starting one. Activities such as painting, dancing, singing, and knitting help boost your sense of self, which can go a long way toward helping you stick with a new way of eating. They also keep you busy, which is important when losing weight. Boredom often leads to only one thing: thoughts about foods you wish you didn't find tempting.

THE YOGA EFFECT

A study of 15,500 men and women determined that study participants who practiced gentle yoga for 30 minutes once a week for 10 years did not gain the typical 2 pounds a year that non-yoga practitioners did. The yoga practitioners who were overweight at the start of the study lost 5 pounds in 10 years, even though they were not dieting. The researchers speculated that increased body awareness allowed study participants to gain more control over their eating choices.

Gentle stretching. The movements we suggest in the following pages will help improve your posture so that your body is better able to withstand the exercise of Programs 2 and 3 without suffering an overuse injury. If you are very overweight, the excess pounds make cardio and other types of exercise painful—and there's no reason to torture yourself. Finally, life has shortened your muscles. If you don't believe us, take a look at any baby or toddler and see how easily they put their toes in their mouths. Can you still do that? We didn't think so. Most of us, over the course of our lives, have stiffened up. That's normal and correctable. This is why we don't want you doing lots of cardio and strength training right now, as both actively shorten muscles. Let's get you flexible first, and then we'll work on your strength.

If you prefer to go to an organized exercise class, sign up for a gentle yoga, stretching, tai chi, or Pilates class. Any of these types of exercise will accomplish your goals of building flexibility and balance.

If you prefer to exercise at home, use this routine three to five times a week.

BALANCE POSE

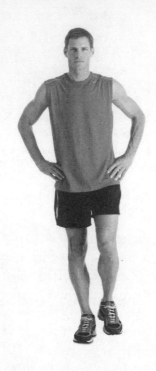

Stand with your feet under your hips. Shift your body weight over your right foot, lifting your left foot an inch or two off the ground. Balance on one foot for up to 30 seconds, tapping your left foot down periodically as needed. Repeat on the right side. Once you can balance for 30 seconds, increase your challenge by doing it with your eyes closed.

DOWN DOG ON TABLE

Stand 2 feet in front of a table. Bend forward at the waist and place your palms against the tabletop. Step back with your feet until your torso forms a right angle with your legs. Reach back through your tailbone and forward through the top of your head, trying to lengthen your spine as much as possible. As you do this, pull up slightly through the navel and downward with your tailbone, to flatten your lower back. Hold for up to 30 seconds and release.

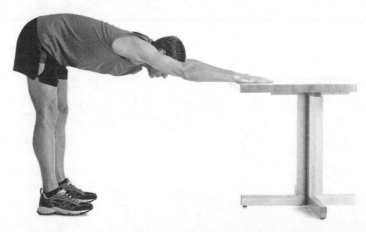

HIP STRETCH

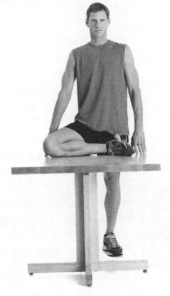

Stand in front of a table. (Your dining room table, bathroom counter, or a desk should work.) If these surfaces are too high, try a stable dining room chair. Place your palms on the surface for support. Lift your right leg and place your right foot, ankle, shin, and knee on the table, lining up your foot and calf with the table's edge. Stand tall and hold. For most people, this is an intense stretch. If you would like to increase the stretch, bend forward at the waist. Hold for up to 30 seconds, and then switch legs and repeat.

SHOULDER STRETCH AND STRENGTHENER

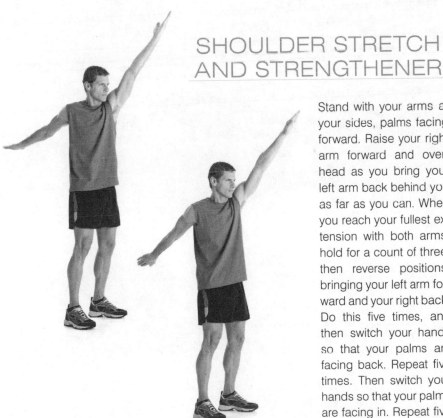

Stand with your arms at your sides, palms facing forward. Raise your right arm forward and overhead as you bring your left arm back behind you as far as you can. When you reach your fullest extension with both arms, hold for a count of three, then reverse positions, bringing your left arm forward and your right back. Do this five times, and then switch your hands so that your palms are facing back. Repeat five times. Then switch your hands so that your palms are facing in. Repeat five times.

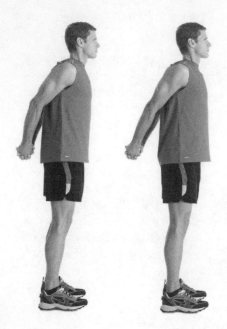

CHEST STRETCH

Stand and clasp your hands behind your back. Roll your shoulders up, back, and down to retract your shoulder blades and lift your breastbone. Reach down through your knuckles until you feel a stretch in your chest and shoulders. To increase the stretch, raise your arms. Hold for up to 30 seconds.

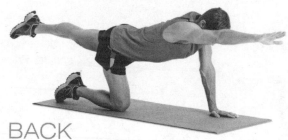

BACK STRENGTHENER

Kneel on all fours with your knees under your hips and your hands under your shoulders. Lift your right arm and left leg, extending both parallel to the floor. Then bring your right elbow and left knee toward one another as you tuck your chin to your chest. Continue to extend and then bend your arm and leg five times. Then switch sides and repeat, using your left arm and right leg.

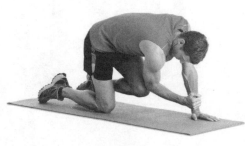

THIGH AND HIP STRETCH

Kneel on your hands and knees. Step your right foot forward, between your hands. Inch your left foot back until you feel a stretch in your thighs and hips. Try to drop down through your pubic bone. You may keep your hands on the floor, or, to increase the stretch, place them on your right thigh and lift your torso upright. Hold for up to 30 seconds, and then switch legs and repeat.

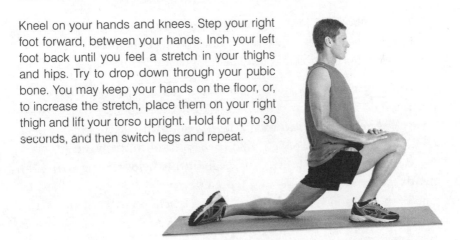

HAMSTRING STRETCH

Lie on your back with your knees bent. Extend your right leg toward the ceiling. Place a bath towel or rope around your foot, clasping the ends of the towel or rope in each hand. Gently use your hands to pull your foot toward your head. Periodically press your foot into the towel or rope, tensing your hamstring for a count of three. This will encourage your hamstring muscle to relax. Stretch for up to 30 seconds. Lower your right leg and repeat with the left leg.

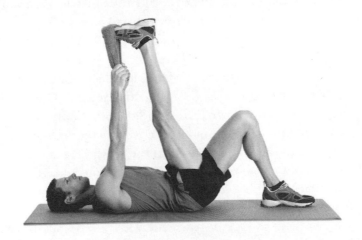

Program 2

Best for:

- People who have lost 5 percent of their initial body weight
- People who feel more energetic since starting the plan
- People who have been on the plan for at least 1 month

You may wonder why we recommend weight lifting in this program rather than cardio. That's a great question and we have a great answer. When it comes to weight loss, weight lifting has an edge over cardio, particularly for people who have an insulin disadvantage.

Many studies have shown that weight lifting helps reverse an insulin disadvantage more quickly and more effectively than cardio does. In one of these studies, completed at the Keck School of Medicine of the University of Southern California in Los Angeles, a twice-a-week weight-lifting program significantly reduced insulin resistance, a condition in which body cells do not respond to insulin, in overweight boys who were genetically prone to developing this problem. This was a permanent, 24-hour-a-day increase in sensitivity that kept insulin levels low and blood sugar steady. Comparatively, research shows that cardio also improves sensitivity, but only for 1 day. That means you would need to do cardio every day to maintain the improvement, whereas strength training gives you the same results in just two weekly sessions—the same number we recommend for the program below.

Why does strength training produce longer-lasting sensitivity? In short, because it builds muscle, and when you increase muscle mass, you increase the number of muscle cells that are available to burn sugar for energy.

We recommend a particular type of weight lifting called SuperSlow. It was developed in 1982 at the University of Florida by a researcher named Ken Hutchins. He used the method to teach older women with osteoporosis how to lift weight safely, without getting injured. Numerous studies completed since have shown that SuperSlow is not only safer than traditional weight lifting but also more effective. It works more muscle fibers, getting you stronger without requiring too much time at the gym. It will take about 10 minutes for Routine 1, 15 to 20 minutes for Routine 2. This includes transition time—moving from one exercise to another.

In the following pages, we provide you with a home-based strength-training workout and a gym-based one. Do the workout in the location that works best for you.

Routine 1

At Home

If you don't feel comfortable working out in front of other people at a gym, you have lots of company. One of the reasons the vast majority of people don't exercise is that they don't feel competent, so they worry what other people will think of them. Use this home workout to build your strength and your confidence.

PUSH-UP

Whether done on your knees or on your toes, the push-up is a great total body strengthener. Place your hands slightly wider than shoulder-distance apart. Tuck your tailbone. Bend your elbows out to the sides as you slowly lower to the floor for 5 seconds. Return to the starting position for 10 seconds. Repeat up to 12 times, stopping and holding for up to 30 seconds on the last push.

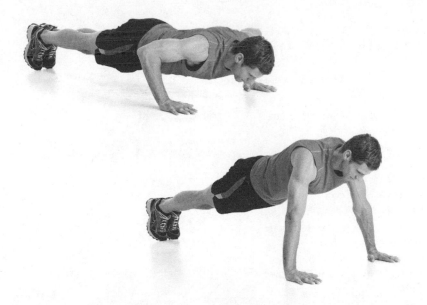

BACK STRENGTHENER

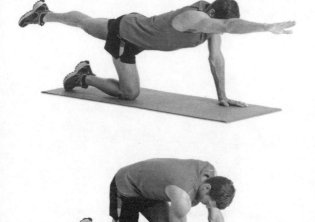

This is the same exercise you did for Program 1, but now we'll add the SuperSlow method to it. Kneel on all fours with your knees under your hips and your hands under your shoulders. Lift your right arm and left leg, taking 10 seconds to extend both parallel to the floor. Then take 5 seconds to bring your right elbow and left knee toward one another as you tuck your chin to your chest. Continue to extend and then bend your arm and leg five times. On the last extension, hold for up to 30 seconds. Then switch sides and repeat, using your left arm and right leg.

SIT BACK

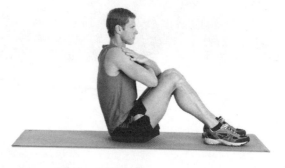

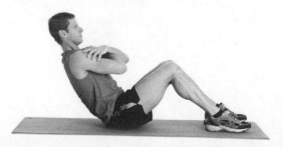

Sit with your knees bent and your feet on the floor. Cross your arms over your chest. Keeping your back flat and your spine extended, sit back as far as you can (until your back is roughly 45 degrees off the floor), taking 10 seconds to move back. Then take 5 seconds to return to the starting position. Repeat up to 12 times.

WALL SQUAT

Stand with your back against a wall. Walk your feet out as you bend your knees, sliding your back down the wall until your legs are bent at right angles. Hold for up to 30 seconds, and then release. Extra credit: If you have a large fitness ball, place it between your back and the wall to improve your balance.

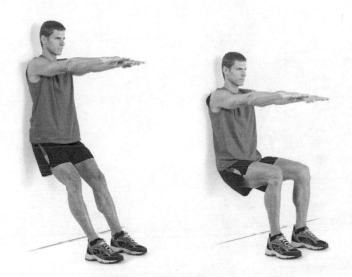

Routine 2

Gym Workout

We recommend using weight machines because you can use heavier weights without risk of injury. Finding the right weight for you will take some trial and error. Don't fret too much about choosing your heaviest weight possible on the first workout. As long as you increase the weight over time, you are getting stronger. Set the weight at something that you feel you can comfortably lift, but that allows you to feel the movement every time. You should struggle to complete the last couple of reps. If the last two reps still feel relatively easy, increase the weight by one plate (5 to 10 pounds) at your next workout. This will challenge more of your muscle fibers, making the workout more effective. The following machines allow you to work large muscle groups, again making your gym time more efficient. If you've never used the machines before, enlist the help of the gym's personal trainer to set them up correctly.

CHEST PRESS

Sit in the machine and adjust the seat so the hand bars are at chest height. Grasp the bars with your palms facing down. Push the bar away from you slowly, taking a full 10 seconds to fully extend your arms. Return to the starting position slowly, taking 5 seconds to do so. Repeat 8 to 12 times.

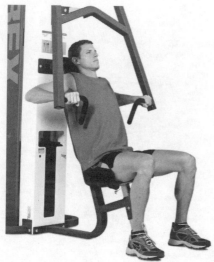

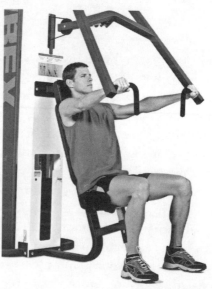

LEG PRESS

Sit in the machine, place your feet on the platform, and adjust the seat so that your knees are bent and your feet are as close to your hips as you can comfortably get them. Press the platform away, taking a full 10 seconds to extend your legs. Return to the starting position and hold for 5 seconds. Repeat 8 to 12 times.

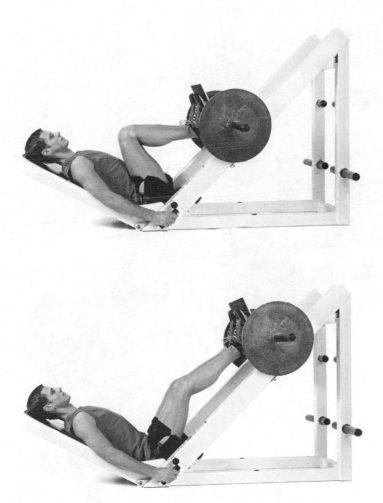

ABDOMINAL MACHINE

Most gyms have some type of abdominal machine. Some machines allow only upper body movement, encouraging you to crunch your upper body toward your legs. Others permit a double crunching motion, moving your upper body downward and your lower body upward. Both are great options. Sit in whichever machine your gym has. Take 10 seconds to crunch and 5 seconds to release. Repeat 8 to 12 times.

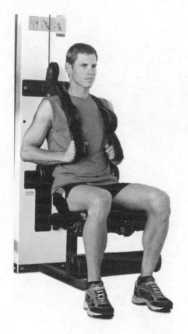

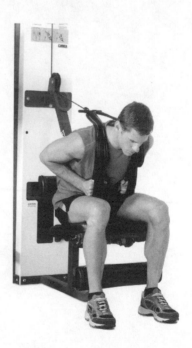

BACK EXTENSION MACHINE

Sit in the machine and put on the seat belt. Push back, taking 10 seconds to extend backward and 5 seconds to return to the starting position. Repeat 8 to 12 times.

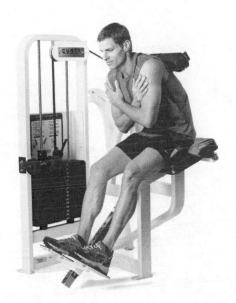

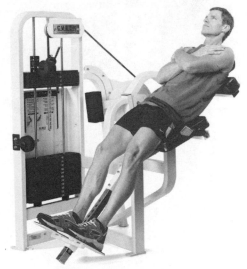

LAT PULLDOWN

Adjust the machine so that your knees fit snugly under the restraint bar. Sit, and grasp the pulldown bar with an underhand grip, placing your hands slightly wider than shoulder width. Take a full 10 seconds to lower the bar to your chest and 5 seconds to return to the starting position. Repeat 8 to 12 times.

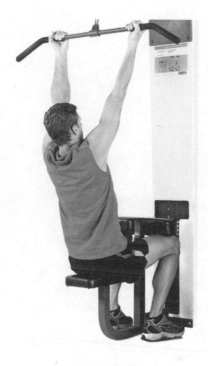

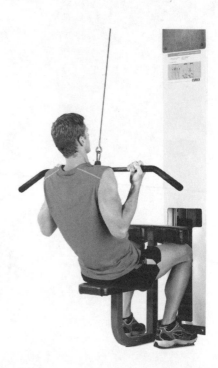

ROW

You'll find two types of rowing machines at most gyms. One involves sitting on an open slab and pulling a cable toward you. In another, you sit with your chest against a restraint and pull two bars toward you. Use either style of rowing machine, taking 10 seconds to row the bar or cable to you and 5 seconds to return to the starting position. Repeat 8 to 12 times.

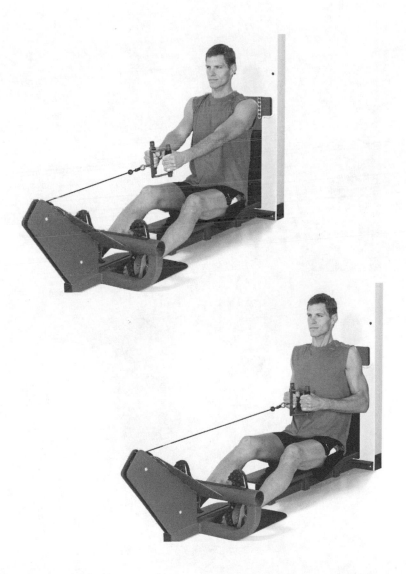

SHOULDER PRESS

Sit in the machine and adjust the seat so that the bars are just over your shoulders. Grasp the bars with an overhand grip. Take 10 seconds to press the bars up and 5 seconds to lower them to the starting position. Repeat 8 to 12 times.

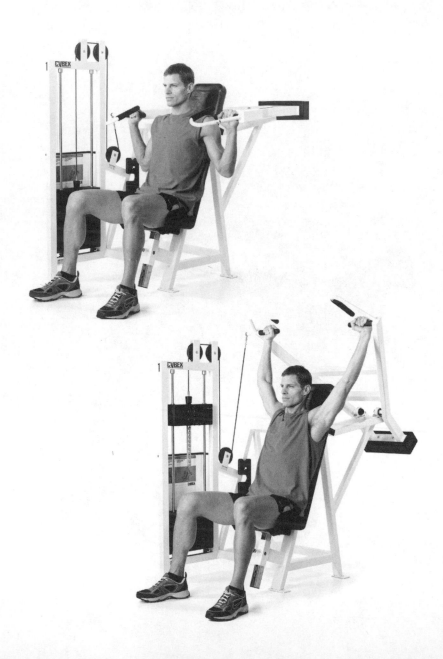

Program 3

Now you're ready to add cardio to the mix. It's very important that you not overdo it. Only progress to Program 3 once:

- You are sleeping well at night
- You no longer feel especially taxed from your Program 2 strengthening workouts
- You feel energetic throughout the day
- You are close to your weight-loss goal

There's no one best way to introduce cardio. Forget about all of the magazine articles promoting the relative merits of a particular piece of cardio equipment. It may be true that intense activities such as running burn more calories than walking, or that whole body movements such as cross-country skiing burn more calories than lower body movements such as stairclimbing, but none of that matters if you hate the type of movement so much that you never do it. You burn fewer calories lying on the couch than you do with any type of movement!

FAMILY FITNESS

Studies show that children become less active with each passing year of their lives. What better way to get motivated to exercise than to move with your children? Here are some ideas:

- Go for family bike rides.

- Have weekly hula hoop contests to see who can keep the hoop going the longest.

- Set up sport cones in the backyard and create fun obstacle course races through the cones. Run backwards, shuttle sideways, or even crawl on all fours. Get creative and have fun.

- Have a "race" night, holding wheelbarrow, three-legged, and other types of races.

- Take turns bouncing on a mini trampoline.

- Do a family yoga video.

- Take a family walk after dinner each night.

- Jump rope.

The best type of cardio is whichever type you like. Rather than think of it as exercise, think of it as movement. Any of the following counts as cardio:

- Playing "Duck, Duck, Goose" and other games with your children
- Walking as you window-shop
- Riding your bike to complete errands such as going to the post office or bank
- Dancing
- Walking on the beach
- Walking the perimeter of the mall before heading into a store
- Taking the stairs

Think about ways to introduce more movement into your life. Perhaps you like the social setting of softball or the solitude of walking on a beach at sunset. Whatever form of movement you choose, make it a positive in your life rather than a negative. Don't use exercise to punish yourself for eating poorly or to burn off the calories you ate for dessert the night before. Use it to get stronger, improve your metabolism, and feel more confident.

If you feel better after moving, then you've pushed yourself well. If you feel tired and achy, you've overdone it. Cardio should give you energy. If it saps you, you're going too long or too intensely. Use this advice to make movement an integral part of your life.

Link it with something you do every day. For example, take a walk after dinner or park farther away from the entrance at work.

Do it with others. If you exercise with someone your age, you may stick with it more easily, according to research done at the University of British Columbia. Make sure your movement partner is equally motivated. If your partner keeps making excuses for not meeting you or suggests you go for coffee instead, it's time to find a new partner.

Set a goal and write it down. Start with 10 minutes of movement a day and work your way up to 20. Carry a small notebook with you, and each time you choose to move—for example, by taking the stairs instead of the elevator—write it down. This record keeping will keep you motivated to continually search out additional ways to sneak in more movement. Once you make a game out of it, it becomes more fun.

KEEP IT OFF

First, let us congratulate you on nearing or reaching your weight-loss goal. You worked hard to get here. We hope that you've seen the difference in more than just your body size. Are you sleeping more soundly? Do you have less gas and bloating? Do you have fewer headaches? How about more energy? Take a moment to savor all of the wonderful physical and emotional changes you've experienced during the past weeks and months. You might even want to write it all down. Doing so will serve as a constant reminder of why you want to keep the weight off and why you want to follow this eating plan for life.

That's what this chapter is all about—providing you with the essentials you need to keep off the weight for good.

Some people assume that once they lose the weight, they can keep it off without staying aware of the food choices they are making. This doesn't work. Thoughtless eating is how you gained the weight in the first place, and it's how you'll regain it if you don't follow a detailed maintenance plan. Let's get something straight right away: You're not done. You never will be. To keep off the weight, you must remain vigilant for the rest of your life.

Got that? The rest of your life.

That's why we just asked you to think about how great you feel at the moment. Remembering how great you feel will go a long way toward helping you stay motivated long term.

Some people go on the diet to lose weight and pledge that they'll keep off the weight by going back to a seemingly "healthier" low-fat diet. They assume there is no way they can continue to eat this much meat, cheese, and other fatty foods and stay healthy. If this is your thought process, we invite you to see for yourself. Go to your primary care doctor as soon as possible for follow-up blood work. If you followed our advice, you got this blood work done before you started the diet and every 3 months as you followed the diet. Now, do it again. If your cholesterol or another health indicator was high during the first checkup, your insurance will probably cover the repeat testing. Call the 800 number listed on your insurance card to see what's covered and what's not. Ask for measurements of your lipid levels, kidney and liver function, blood sugar, insulin levels, blood pressure, and other markers of good health. We're convinced that you'll learn that they have all improved since you started eating our way.

If that's not enough to put your worried mind at rest, go ahead and get health tests regularly. If you experience increases in cholesterol, blood pressure, or blood glucose, okay, maybe you need to modify something. Maybe you need to cut back on red meat, butter, cream, and cheese (the sources of saturated fat most likely to raise cholesterol) and focus on consuming fat from plant foods (olives, olive oil, coconut oil, avocados, flaxseed, nuts, and cocoa) and fish.

We're almost certain, however, that your numbers are not going to go up. We know because we've worked with hundreds of people who used this eating approach not only to lose weight but also to keep it off long term while improving their health and reducing overall body aging. We're convinced that it's the healthiest way to eat. If we weren't, we wouldn't both still be following the fundamentals of the diet years after we've each lost weight.

BEFORE YOU REACH YOUR GOAL

About 4 to 6 weeks before you believe you'll reach your goal, start thinking about maintenance. Gradually change your mind-set from restricting foods in order to lose weight to following a healthful, balanced diet. Do this by adding foods back into your culinary repertoire. Start adding carbohydrate foods back in, using as guidance the serving suggestions and suggested foods from the eating plans outlined in Chapters 6 through 8. Add a new food every week or two, noticing how you feel as you incorporate it. This is especially important if you had a yeast disadvantage, because certain foods may irritate your GI

Q: *If my LDL cholesterol goes up, should I switch to a low-fat diet?*

A: Most of our patients experience a dramatic improvement in their cholesterol levels, with a decrease in triglycerides, VLDL, and LDL levels, as well as an increase in the good HDL levels. More important, their LDL and HDL particle sizes increase, making the LDL less dangerous and the HDL more protective. You want your ratio of total cholesterol to HDL (total cholesterol divided by HDL) below 4 and, ideally, closer to 2.

A minority of people experience a temporary rise in LDL and total cholesterol because the body sometimes releases cholesterol as it releases fat. This rise is usually in the good type of LDL (large particle size or pattern A). As we've mentioned earlier, it's small, dense LDL particles that raise heart disease risk. In this minority of patients, LDL usually comes down in 3 to 6 months as the body burns through its fat stores. This probably isn't anything to be worried about. If your LDL rises, ask your physician to do more detailed blood work that breaks down your type of LDL. Our diet should change your LDL into a more desirable type (large particle size) that is not as likely to gum up your arteries.

If you find that the small, dense type of LDL (called LDL particle type B) goes up, then reduce carbs first. Keep a 5-day food diary to see whether refined or sweetened foods have crept back into your diet. If they haven't, then cut back on red meat, butter, cream, and cheese, opting to consume most of your fat from plant foods and fish. You don't, however, have to go low fat. Doing so may worsen cholesterol even more.

---

tract. Adding one new food at a time will help you pinpoint which foods trigger bloating and gas.

The week or two before you reach your goal, you should be eating all of the foods we mentioned in the "Maintenance Is as Easy as 1-2-3" section on page 143, including legumes, whole grain bread and crackers, fruit, and more. Your weight loss will slow as you progress to this balanced way of eating. That's normal. In fact, some people are so masterful at adding foods back in that, when they reach their goal weight, they automatically stop losing. They are eating their maintenance diet!

AFTER YOU REACH YOUR GOAL

You will need to remain conscious of your eating choices for the rest of your life. You don't, however, have to eat 100 percent healthy all the time. Most of the time, eat real foods: eggs, meat, vegetables, fruit, whole grains, legumes, and so on. Some of the time, splurge. It's okay to enjoy ice cream every once in a while. It's okay to savor a chocolate chip cookie or a small slice of pie. It's okay as long as you hold yourself to a reasonable portion and stay in control as you eat.

How do you stay in control? Test yourself. Do not be afraid to take this important step. You may have more control than you think. You have weaned yourself off sugar. You have changed your taste preferences. Your brain isn't used to having so much sugar, so your tolerance for it is lower. You no longer have yeast and insulin disadvantages and other problems that trigger cravings for sweets. Your body is also working more efficiently. Case in point: One of our diabetic patients found that after she'd lost 7 pounds by following the Level 1 and Level 2 eating plans, she could eat two squares of 72 percent chocolate, ⅓ cup of whole grains, half a sweet potato, or one slice of flax bread and have it hardly affect her blood sugar. She had improved her body's efficiency, so these foods no longer dramatically spiked her blood sugar.

Keep in mind that ice cream and other dessert foods are usually high in saturated fat and sugar. These will never become "all you can eat" foods. Feeling in control is critical to feeling comfortable.

MAUREEN WELLINGTON LOST 12 POUNDS!

This is the only diet that works for me. I just needed a little guidance and motivation to get myself to do it. The Berkowitzes handed me a list of food recommendations, and I follow it. I've lost 2½ to 3 inches all over my body. This weight loss is costing me a small fortune in alterations. I feel so much better, too. My blood pressure and blood sugar are down.

Since I committed myself to the plan, I have not had any cake, pie, or ice cream. Do I miss them? No; I'm better off if I don't eat sweets. I keep them out of the house. I now watch everything that goes in my mouth. I'm more aware of eating, and I reach for real foods rather than processed foods. It's a healthy lifestyle, bottom line.

How often can you indulge? The answer to that question depends on many factors, including your confidence level. Some people settle into a rhythm in which they find they can manage an indulgence once a day. Others can do so only once a week, and still others can do so only once a month. In addition to your confidence level, your personal prescription depends on your body size (taller, more muscular people can generally get away with eating more carbs than shorter, thin-boned, less muscular people can), gender (men can usually eat more carbs than women can), age (younger people can usually get away with eating more carbs than older people can) genetics, and metabolic health (a thyroid disadvantage requires a delicate balance; an insulin disadvantage or diabetes means you must eat fewer carbs than someone who does not have these conditions). Regular strength training and cardiovascular exercise will allow you to eat more carbs, too.

To indulge in sweet treats and other foods every once in a while—without losing control or regaining weight—follow this advice.

Stay within 3 to 5 pounds of your final destination. If the scale goes up 3 pounds, take a step back and look at what you are doing. Don't let 3 pounds turn into 6, and 6 turn into 12. It could be water weight, but it could also be a sign that you are gaining. Return to keeping a food diary and look at how you've been eating. If you start to gain, cut back until you can maintain.

Avoid trigger foods. Valerie recently counseled a patient who mentioned that he and his wife have completely different experiences when they eat brownies. He gets a rush when he eats sugar, losing control and eating more than he would like to, whereas his wife savors every bite and is satisfied after just one brownie.

If you feel out of control when you eat certain foods, avoid those foods. You need to feel in control, and right now, you are afraid of losing control. Don't reintroduce foods that cause you to lose control. For you, eating a little bit of those foods is like an alcoholic having a little bit of beer or a former smoker trying to stop at just one butt. Continue to avoid foods that:

- Cause you to feel ashamed or disgusted after eating
- You eat more rapidly than other foods
- You tend to eat past an uncomfortable fullness
- You tend to eat in large amounts when you are not really hungry

Try to be realistic. We all travel. We all attend dinners at friends' homes, where choices may be tempting. Remember: It's your choice, and you can remain in control. We all indulge from time to time. As long as you keep those indulgences to a minimum, you will be able to keep off the weight. Don't stress about occasional luxuries. Stress is just as bad for your metabolism as poor eating habits are.

Follow the one indulgence rule. Stick with your eating plan most of the time, indulging every once in a while in a balanced and controlled way. For instance, if you go out to eat, the core of your meal will always be the same. Start with a salad and as your main course have meat or fish with 2 cups of vegetables. Then have one indulgence. It might be an appetizer, a glass of wine, or sharing a small dessert with a dining companion. It's not all three. For instance, if you are at a wedding, you can have one or two pastry puffs, one or two pigs in a blanket, one alcoholic beverage, *or* the piece of wedding cake. Don't have all of them.

Eat wholesome foods first. It's okay to indulge from time to time, but it's not okay to indulge during every single meal and snack. If you notice you are craving dessert simply because you are hungry, satisfy your craving with real food first. Have a burger patty or tuna salad. If your taste for indulging is still there, go for it. If not, you won—and the victory will be reflected in your weight.

When in doubt, eat real food. If you want to indulge in something sweet, do so, but make it a small serving of a real food. Ice cream means sugar and cream, and almost nothing else. Don't go for the low-fat or artificially sweetened varieties. These are not only less satisfying and satiating, but they also tend to cause people to lose self-control. It's psychological. When we eat reduced-calorie foods, we assume we can have more. When we eat high-calorie foods, we assume we can have less and stick to it.

Beware of change. Any life change—a new job, new responsibilities at work, the purchase of a new home, a new baby—can be a catalyst for weight gain. It's so easy, when we're under stress, to revert to bad habits. Even if you backslide a little during a stressful time, get back on track as soon as possible. If you've gained a little weight, drop down to the basic plan of Level 2 or Level 1 until you lose it, and then recommit to your maintenance plan.

STAY COMMITTED

Now you know almost everything you need to know to lose all the weight you want and keep it off for good. We've added this final chapter, however, because we've worked with enough dieters over the years to know that weight loss really isn't about food, and it isn't about exercise. It's about change. It's about forming new habits, and it's about confronting all of the varied excuses that can easily tempt you to abandon your hard efforts. Excuses such as fatigue, bad breath, or constantly feeling deprived.

We have great news for you. You can overcome all of these excuses! We hope you use the following advice to motivate yourself toward success.

BACKSLIDING

Everyone backslides. You might slip up as early as the first week of the diet, or it might not happen until the first month, the sixth month, or even 6 months after reaching your goal weight. But at some point, it will happen. An old bad habit will creep back into your daily nutritional repertoire. It might be the bagel you used to enjoy each morning for breakfast. It might be pizza on a Friday night. Instead of holding yourself to one vegetable-loaded slice of thin crust, for example, you go overboard with three or four slices with extra cheese. It might be that you find yourself continually dishing up larger servings than you should be eating.

Whatever it is, the first slip can easily lead to more slips, which can lead to a plateau, which can lead to gaining. If you don't put the brakes on this cycle, you can easily find yourself back where you started—regaining all of the pounds you lost, and then some.

Just ask David Schipper. He came to Valerie 3 months before his wedding. He weighed 231 pounds, had high triglycerides, and was insulin resistant. He didn't know it at the time, but his carbohydrate-rich eating style and excess pounds were contributing to low energy levels, higher stress levels, insomnia, and GI discomfort. He readily followed the diet we prescribed, and the pounds dropped off—fast. In just 12 weeks he lost 33 pounds, shedding 5 inches from his waist. His triglycerides and insulin returned to normal. He started sleeping better at night. He told us he handled stress better at work. His GI distress resolved. He reached his goal weight, and he kept it off for 6 months. He was one of our proudest success stories.

That is, until we learned that he had regained the weight. "It was a slow transition back to the dark side," he told us. "It started with a bagel here and a cookie there. After a couple of months of these indiscretions, I was back eating the way I had before I lost the weight. Then I gained the weight back."

How does someone who seems to have mastered the lifestyle backslide so quickly? The reasons differ from person to person, but they generally have a common theme. David admits he slowly gave up his new healthy habits, putting old weight-gaining habits in their place. Here's how we got David and others like him back on track.

Create serving-size cues. It's easy to tell yourself that you will hold yourself to ½ cup of fruit, one slice of bread, one scoop of ice cream, or one cracker. It's another thing to do it. The one scoop of ice cream turns into half of the container. The cracker turns into a third of the package. The bread turns into a sandwich, or two.

Studies show that, when it comes to appetite control, size matters. Most of us eat more from larger bowls than from smaller bowls, for example. We drink more from wider glasses than from narrower glasses. We also tend to eat more from containers—the bag of chips, the ice cream carton, the raisin container—than we would if we took food out of the container and placed it on a plate before eating.

Case in point: In a study at the University of Illinois, graduate students attended a lecture about how large serving bowls induce overeating. They then went to a Super Bowl party. Those who scooped Chex mix from larger serving bowls put 55 percent more onto their plates than those who reached for the same amount of mix from a smaller serving bowl. Other studies show that we do the same with popcorn, eating more from a large container than from a small one. This is true even if the popcorn is 14 days old and incredibly stale. If the container is big, we shovel the food into our mouths, even if the food doesn't taste all that great!

Research also shows that we tend to eat food more quickly when we see more. In a study at the University of Rhode Island, women who were given a plate of pasta and a big spoon slurped down 646 calories of pasta in 9 minutes. When they were given a small serving of pasta and a small spoon, they took up to 30 minutes to eat and consumed fewer calories.

You can use this research to provide yourself with extra control when it comes to the carbohydrate foods you love.

- When serving grains, use appetizer plates (about 4 inches in diameter) instead of dinner plates.
- When serving yourself fruit, use fruit cups, coffee cups (note: we're referring to the old-fashioned cups that come with saucers and not the newfangled mugs that hold a quart of liquid), or a small child's bowl instead of regular-size bowls.
- Put wine and other types of alcohol in a tall, skinny glass rather than in a short, wide one.
- Dish all food onto a plate before eating, so you can easily see your portion size. Never eat anything straight from a container or bag.

These simple tricks provide an optical illusion. Your brain thinks you are eating or drinking more, when you are really eating or drinking less. End result: You feel more satisfied on fewer carbohydrates.

Break old habits. Our bodies signal us to eat based on our usual eating habits. You get hungry at 8 a.m. because you usually eat at 8 a.m. Same with lunchtime. Same with dinner. If you snack at midafternoon, you'll start to get hungry for your snack around the time you usually eat it. If you decide not to snack or have a meal at a given time, your body will still expect the snack, and even if you are not physically hungry, you can get a case of pseudo-hunger where you feel hungry even if you just ate 20 minutes earlier!

This habitual hunger, by the way, also works in reverse. Studies show that skipping one meal regularly will cause less ghrelin to be released at that specific mealtime. If you want to stop feeling hungry for a bedtime snack, all you have to do is go a few nights without it.

The same goes for sights, sounds, and smells that surround eating. You will constantly think about food in specific trigger situations that you have associated with eating. For example, many people want to eat when they watch television because they have always done so. If you have a particular affinity for specific carbohydrate foods, take a moment to think about the places and situations where you tend to eat those foods. For David Schipper, driving past Dunkin' Donuts was all it took for him to think about backsliding into his first bagel. Which people, places, situations, and events make you think about bread, cereal, fruit, dessert, and other carbohydrate foods? Think about how you can change your daily routine to avoid those triggers. If you change your routine enough, you'll be less likely to backslide because the cues won't be there to tempt you. Below are some ideas that have worked for our clients in specific situations.

Problem: You are tempted by pizza and other foods served at business meetings.

Solution: Go to the meeting with alternative foods in hand. Perhaps take some nuts, a mozzarella stick, or raw veggies with blue cheese dressing. You can also try strengthening your resolve by eating before the meeting, so you are not tempted to have the pizza. If it's just a periodic meeting, go with a strategy. Perhaps you eat the cheese off the pizza and have a salad, or you have just one small slice of pizza.

Problem: You're tempted to eat starchy carbs whenever your young children are eating macaroni and cheese, grilled cheese, or noodles.

Solution: First, your children's health is just as important as yours, right? Serve them healthier versions of these foods. Make grilled cheese with whole grain, low-carb bread. Use whole grain pasta for macaroni and cheese. Make both dishes occasional once-a-week treats rather than everyday occurrences. It may be hard to believe, but your children really will not starve to death when deprived of macaroni and cheese. When they get hungry enough, they will eat whatever you put in front of them.

Problem: You don't have time for breakfast, so you end up eating a muffin or bagel later when you feel hungry.

Solution: Stash breakfast options at work, in the car, or wherever you find you are tempted by high-carbohydrate convenience foods. For instance, keep Wasa crackers with cream cheese or almond butter at work. Make a dozen hard-boiled eggs at the beginning of each week and stash them in the break room mini fridge to eat as needed. Eat easy but nontraditional breakfast options, such as turkey wrapped with cheese and some sliced avocado.

Problem: You tend to reach for something sugary in the midafternoon because you are so hungry you could eat your own arm.

Solution: Eat a vegetable, protein, or protein/fat snack an hour before you usually get hungry. Try raw vegetables dipped in hummus or guacamole. Another great option is cottage or ricotta cheese mixed with a teaspoon of almond butter. You can also order or make a larger than usual lunch, eating half for lunch and the other half in the midafternoon.

FATIGUE

You may experience some fatigue during the first few days of the diet, as your body switches from a carbohydrate metabolism to a fat metabolism. Most of the people we work with report amazing energy levels after a week or two of following the food plan. In fact, one man told us he felt so energetic within a week of starting the diet that he was running full speed uphill—for the fun of it.

This energy also comes from your body's newfound ability to burn fat for fuel, sparing muscle glycogen. Your body has a near endless supply of fat but a very limited supply of stored carbohydrate. This switch

EAT FAT TO RUN FAST

A study at the University of Buffalo determined that runners who switched from a low-fat diet to a high-fat diet for 2 months improved their running performance. Additional research at the same institution has shown that endurance athletes who restrict fat tend to experience a drop in immunity and an increase in the incidence of colds and flu. According to the researchers, a diet too low in fat increases levels of pro-inflammatory cytokines (a type of immune system chemical) and free radicals and inhibits levels of anti-inflammatory cytokines. Adding more fat can increase levels of important immune cells that fight infection. Finally, when runners ate more fat, there was no ill effect on their weight, blood pressure, or cholesterol levels.

to a fat metabolism, theoretically, should equip you with more endurance and more energy, not less. In fact, research shows that endurance athletes who switch to a very low-carbohydrate, very high-fat diet do not lose their endurance. Some studies show that they can even last longer without feeling fatigued.

So why are you so tired? If you are still feeling fatigued after one or two weeks, it may be due to any of the following factors.

Dehydration. When you switch to a fat metabolism, you will lose a lot of body water. Your body stores water with glycogen (the stored form of carbohydrate). During the first week of the diet, your body will burn through these glycogen stores, releasing lots of water into your urine. Take extra precautions to stay hydrated. Drink at least six to eight 8-ounce glasses of water, evenly spacing them throughout the day.

Mineral loss. As you shed water during the first week of this eating plan, you'll also lose minerals. Make sure you are taking the supplements we recommended in Chapter 9. In particular, you may feel low in energy if you are low in either calcium or magnesium.

Stress. If you have functioned with high levels of cortisol for a long period of time, you may find that you feel drained when cortisol levels return to normal. We call this the vacation effect, as many of our patients had told us that they felt drained and slept 10 or more hours every day when they were on vacation. If you have depleted your adrenals, it may take longer for your energy levels to return. Take it easy. Do not exercise and try to rest as much as you can.

CONSTIPATION

Some people claim that low-carb diets cause constipation. This may be true with some types of low-carb diets, because many of their meal plans are notoriously low in fiber. It is true of ours only if you don't follow the plan as directed! Many of our patients find that when they follow the diet correctly, their constipation, gas, and other GI complaints resolve. If yours do not, or if you become constipated, try the following.

Eat more vegetables. Most vegetables are low in carbohydrates and rich in fiber. Their fiber score is above 75 percent. The fiber in vegetables and other plant foods gets things moving by increasing the weight and size of feces. As fiber travels through the digestive tract, it absorbs water, which softens and adds bulk to stool. This speeds and

ARE YOU CONSTIPATED?

You should have one or two easy-to-pass stools a day. By "easy-to-pass," we mean that you sit down, you relax, and you go. You do not have time to read the paper, a novel, or a magazine. If this does not describe you, you are probably constipated.

eases the passage of stool through the colon. Fiber may also trigger muscles along the sides of the intestines to contract and relax (called peristalsis), helping push stool along.

Are you consuming at least 3 cups of leafy and green vegetables and 2 cups of other vegetables daily? If not, make an effort to do so. Use these pointers.

- Purchase plastic food containers in various cup sizes. Fill these containers with salad greens or chopped veggies and take them with you for an easy lunch or snack. This allows you to easily know how many cups you've gotten in during a given day.
- Precede lunch and dinner with a salad. Starting your meal with a salad provides the side benefit of filling you up, so you are less tempted to reach for the bread or pasta.
- Buy an assortment of frozen vegetables. Many of these will steam in the bag, making them quick and easy to prepare. Serve one every night with dinner.

Drink more water. Fiber absorbs water as it passes through the GI tract. If you don't drink enough water, your stool grows in size from the fiber, but it dries out and hardens, causing constipation and gas. Get a 25-ounce bottle, fill it each morning, and carry it with you. Drink four a day.

Eat more fat. Fat lubricates the lining of the intestines, allowing stool to pass more easily. If you are eating enough fiber and drinking plenty of water, consider adding olive oil to salads, eating avocado daily, and mixing ground flaxseed into whatever you are eating.

Take magnesium. Magnesium is a natural laxative. If the above strategies do not get things moving, consider taking 500 to 1,000 milligrams of magnesium oxide at night before bed. (Don't use magnesium if you have any kidney problems.)

Q: *Should I take a fiber supplement?*

A: In a word, no. Are you surprised? Many of our patients are. They stare at us with eyes the size of dinner plates when we tell them to stop using their supplemental fiber. The fiber supplement industry has done its advertising and marketing so well that nearly everyone in America is convinced they need to drop some powder in a glass of water, stir, and drink every morning. It's just not true.

In fact, you might be surprised to learn that most fiber supplements contain very little fiber. Most foods contain more. Take a look at the nutrition facts panel on any fiber supplement. You'll find that most supplements contain somewhere between 3 and 5 grams of fiber and 25 or so calories. You can easily get that much fiber from food. More important, the fiber in food comes in a complete package that aids digestion. A colleague of ours at Johns Hopkins Hospital, Gerard E. Mullin, MD, director of Integrative GI Nutrition Services, tells us that nearly all of his patients who take fiber supplements experience lots of gas and bloating and little constipation relief. Real foods work better, he says, because most contain water and/or oil, two essential ingredients that help fiber do its job.

Q: *How can I tell whether I have bad breath?*

A: If a loved one tells you, believe it. What if you live alone and don't want to inflict a breath test on a friend or coworker? Try this simple self-test. It's not completely reliable, but it's the best test around short of breathing into someone else's face.

1. Lick the back of your hand.
2. Let the saliva dry.
3. Smell the back of your hand.

If your hand smells, chances are your breath does, too.

BAD BREATH

As your body burns fat, it creates by-products called ketones. Your body can burn these for energy, but it can also release them through your urine, sweat, and breath. Unfortunately, they can sometimes be a little stinky.

Critics of low-carb diets claim that only this type of diet results in ketone-induced bad breath. This simply isn't true. If you are losing weight, then you are burning fat, and if you are burning fat, your body is making ketones. On a low-carb diet, you are likely burning more fat, so the ketone side effects are more noticeable. Try these remedies.

Drink a lot of water. It will dilute the ketones, reducing their smelly punch.

Chew on parsley, basil, or cilantro. Season your foods with these spices as well. They are all rich sources of chlorophyll, the green pigment in plants that enables photosynthesis.

EMOTIONAL EATING

Do you eat when you are under stress? How about when you feel sad or angry? Although emotional eating is very common—among men and women—it's also destructive. In fact, it's the main reason David Schipper, the dieter we mentioned earlier in this chapter, regained his weight. After losing 33 pounds and keeping it off for 6 months, he took on more responsibility at work. The longer hours and stressful deadlines had him dreaming of bagels and cookies.

To overcome emotional eating—whether you eat out of stress, sadness, anxiety, or even happiness—you must break the association that links your emotional state with eating.

First, get honest with yourself. There's probably a little voice inside your head that's whispering phrases such as "But I'm really hungry," "But I really need it," or "But I can't stop myself." Oh, hush. True hunger comes on slowly. You can satisfy true hunger with any food, including broccoli. Emotional hunger surfaces quickly and centers on one or two specific foods. With emotional hunger, broccoli or a meatball won't do. You must have the bread or bagel or cake or cookie or whatever it is that calls to you.

As soon as you realize that you are craving a specific food, you need to find a way to soothe yourself with something other than food. Think back to the alternative nonfood-related activities we suggested in Chapter 5. Now is the time to employ them.

Think about which emotions drive you to eat. Then think about other ways you can deal with those emotions. Use these ideas to get started.

Sadness: Call a friend. Watch a funny or uplifting movie. Watch a humorous YouTube video. Walk outdoors. Sit outdoors and listen to the sounds of wildlife or of children playing.

Anxiety: Exercise. Walk outdoors. Call a friend. Learn meditation, progressive muscle relaxation, yoga, deep breathing, or another form of relaxation. Listen to a relaxation CD. Read a novel. Pet a dog or cat. Ask a friend or loved one to give you a massage. Take a bath.

Happiness/Celebration: Hug a loved one. Do a victory dance or, better yet, go dancing. Go shopping. Splurge on tickets to a show.

These are just some ideas. We encourage you to come up with your own. Get a piece of paper and list many ideas. Then try them. You may find that some work better than others, and that some work some of the time but not at other times. That's why you have a list! If you try one strategy but still feel the call of food, move on to the next strategy on the list.

If, despite your list, you still find yourself reaching for the cake, tell yourself, "Okay, I'm allowed to have this, but not until I do the following three things." Stop yourself from eating and follow these steps:

1. **Create a weight loss Progress Report and carry it with you.** It doesn't have to be fancy. Some notes jotted down on a piece of paper will do. Write down how much you've lost and any side benefits you've noticed. Feeling more energetic? Write it down. Has your mood improved? Write it down. Have you been able to reduce your dosages of specific medications or stop taking them altogether? Definitely write it down! Are you physically able to accomplish tasks you were not able to accomplish before you lost weight? Write it down. Think of as much as you can, and jot it down on your Progress Report. Add to it over time.

   Whenever you are tempted to eat emotionally, pull it out and read it out loud. Some of our patients find that it helps to read the report before typical tough times during the day—times when they are usually tempted to eat emotionally.

2. **Remind yourself of how terrible you are going to feel after overeating carbs.** Will you end up with a carb hangover? Probably. You may end up getting a headache, feeling lethargic, or any number of other undesirable symptoms. Plus, you'll feel guilty and bad about yourself for deviating from your diet.

3. **Close your eyes and focus your attention inward.** Notice your thoughts and feelings. How do you feel? What thoughts are running through your mind? Why are you turning to the bagel, the cake, or the ice cream? Get in touch with these feelings. Why do you feel this way? What is the problem that triggered these feelings? Are you dissatisfied with your relationship? Is something going wrong with your career? Are you annoyed with a friend? Ask yourself, "What am I really hungry for?" Start problem solving. Solve the problem that is making you feel this way.

If, after going through this three-step process, you still want the cookie, then eat it. **But eat it slowly.** Smell it. Savor it. Taste every bite. Chew every bite thoroughly. Be completely in the moment as you eat.

Then write it down. **Get out that food diary or piece of paper and write down what you ate.** This makes you accountable and helps stop you from reaching for a second or third cookie.

Then forgive yourself. **You strayed.** You ate the cookie. So what? Get right back on the diet and promise yourself that next time, you'll go for a walk rather than eat the cookie.

There. Now you really do know everything you need to know to lose weight and keep it off. You know that many carbs are not your friend—but fiber is. You know that eating fat can help you lose fat. And you know that the trick to heading off cravings is building in a pressure valve, a "cheat release" that allows you to have the foods you want when you need them most. You have all the knowledge you need to maintain a lifelong nutritional plan that will help prevent diabetes, heart disease, cancer, and other serious chronic illnesses. And you can do it all while having some ice cream, bread, wine, and chocolate. Kinda the best of all worlds, huh? We thought you'd agree.

We're so proud of you for taking on this important challenge. We wish you the best of luck. You can do this. Remember to eat early, and eat often. Whenever you stumble, pick yourself back up. You may stumble and fall many times. But as long as you continually get back up and dust off those knees, nothing can stop you from reaching your goal.

RECIPES

LEVEL 1 AND LEVEL 2 RECIPES

You may use the following recipes whether you are following Level 1 or Level 2.

Garden Omelet

1 tablespoon unsalted butter
¼ cup sliced mushrooms
¼ large tomato, diced
3 eggs, beaten
¼ cup chopped baby spinach
1 ounce shredded cheese (any type)

Heat the butter in an omelet pan or a small skillet over medium heat. Add the mushrooms. Cook until the mushrooms soften, 2 to 3 minutes. Add the tomato and eggs. As soon as the eggs start to set, after about 20 seconds, add the spinach. Pat down the spinach with the back of a spatula. Once the spinach starts to wilt, after about 30 seconds, add the cheese. Cook for 2 minutes longer, or until the omelet sets. Fold and serve.

Makes 1 serving

Grilled Cheese

1 tablespoon coconut oil

1 tablespoon unsalted butter

2 slices Alvarado Street bread*

¼ tomato, thinly sliced

½ cup baby spinach

2 slices any cheese

Heat the oil in a skillet over medium heat.

Spread the butter on one side of each slice of bread. Place the tomato, spinach, and cheese between the slices. (Wedge the spinach between the cheese slices, because the cheese will wilt the spinach as it melts.) Place in the pan and cook until each side is brown and the cheese melts, about 5 minutes.

Makes 1 serving

French Toast

1 tablespoon coconut oil

2 eggs

1 teaspoon vanilla extract

2 slices Alvarado Street bread*

Pinch of cinnamon

2 tablespoons chopped walnuts

Heat the oil in a skillet over medium heat.

Beat the eggs and vanilla in a small bowl. Dip each slice of bread into the egg mixture, thoroughly coating the bread, and then sprinkle each side with cinnamon and dip into the walnuts. Place in the heated pan and cook until each side is golden brown, about 1 or 2 minutes per side.

Makes 1 serving

*In Level 2, you can use any of the recommended breads, though only the Alvarado Street brand is appropriate for Level 1.

Vanilla Almond Smoothie

This counts as a higher carbohydrate fruit option.

1 cup unsweetened vanilla-flavored almond milk
1 tablespoon Greens + Wild Berry Burst juice
1 tablespoon vanilla-flavored whey protein
1 teaspoon flaxseed oil
1 teaspoon vanilla extract
½ cup frozen strawberries

Put the almond milk, juice, whey protein, flaxseed oil, vanilla, and strawberries into a blender. Blend until smooth. Serve immediately.

Makes 1 serving

Spinach and Feta Omelet

1 tablespoon unsalted butter
3 eggs, beaten
¾ cup chopped baby spinach
1 ounce crumbled feta cheese

Melt the butter in an omelet pan or a small skillet over medium heat. Add the eggs. As soon as the eggs start to set, about 20 seconds, add the spinach. Pat down the spinach with the back of a spatula. Once the spinach starts to wilt, after about 30 seconds, add the feta. Cook for 2 minutes longer, or until the omelet sets. Fold and serve.

Makes 1 serving

Eggs Florentine

    1 tablespoon unsalted butter
  10 ounces frozen chopped spinach, thawed
        Salt and pepper
    6 eggs

Preheat the oven to 350°F.

Melt the butter in an omelet pan or a small skillet over medium heat. Add the spinach, mixing thoroughly. Season with salt and pepper to taste. Set aside.

Coat a standard 6-cup muffin pan with nonstick spray and add 1 tablespoon of water to each cup. Break 1 egg into each cup. Bake for 15 to 20 minutes.

Arrange the spinach in 6 small mounds on a platter. Place 1 egg on top of each pile of spinach.

Makes 3 servings

Strawberry Sensation Smoothie

When made with plain yogurt, this smoothie will taste somewhat sour. Some people don't mind that flavor. If you do, then consider adding ½ to 1 teaspoon of real vanilla extract or the optional stevia. This recipe was adapted from the book *Are Your Kids Running on Empty?* by Ellen Briggs and Sally Byrd. This smoothie counts as a higher carbohydrate fruit option.

    ½ cup unsweetened plain 2% Greek yogurt
    ½ cup strawberries
    ½ teaspoon almond extract
        Dash of cinnamon
        Dash of stevia (optional)
        Ice cubes

Put the yogurt, strawberries, almond extract, cinnamon, stevia (if using), and ice cubes in a blender. Blend until smooth. Serve immediately.

Makes 1 serving

Michelle's Relaxing Mocktail

½ cup vegetable juice
1 teaspoon horseradish
1 teaspoon hot sauce

Put the vegetable juice, horseradish, and hot sauce in an 8-ounce glass. Stir vigorously, and serve.

Makes 1 serving

Sharon's Chocolate Dream

4 tablespoons sugar-free chocolate syrup
4 tablespoons unsweetened almond milk
¾ cup zero-carb seltzer

Put the syrup, almond milk, and seltzer in an 8-ounce glass, one at a time. Stir to combine, and serve.

Makes 1 serving

Herb Frittata with Cremini Mushrooms and Goat Cheese

1 tablespoon coconut oil

6 eggs

1 tablespoon chopped fresh tarragon plus 1 sprig for garnish

1 tablespoon chopped chives

Dash of milk

Sea or kosher salt and pepper

2 tablespoons unsalted butter

2 cups sliced cremini mushrooms

1 tablespoon chopped scallions

1 ounce crumbled goat cheese or freshly grated Parmigiano-Reggiano

Preheat the oven to 350°F. Lightly coat a 10" ovenproof skillet with the coconut oil. Set aside.

In a medium bowl, whisk together the eggs, 1 tablespoon of tarragon, chives, milk, and salt and pepper to taste.

Melt 1 tablespoon of the butter in the skillet over medium heat. Add the mushrooms and scallions, stirring to coat with the melted butter. Add the remaining 1 tablespoon of butter. Cook, stirring constantly, for 2 minutes, or until the mushrooms are soft and brown. Add the egg mixture. Reduce the heat to low. Cook for 2 minutes, or until the edges of the egg turn opaque and solid. Use a spatula to gently separate the edge of the frittata from the side of the pan to check for doneness. Remove from the heat.

Sprinkle the goat cheese on top of the frittata. Bake for 5 to 6 minutes, or until the eggs are only slightly runny in the middle. Increase the heat to broil and cook for 2 minutes, or until the frittata rises and the top is golden brown. Remove from the oven. Serve with the sprig of fresh tarragon.

Makes 4 servings

Guacamole

5 ripe avocados

1 medium red onion, chopped

2 jalapeño chile peppers, seeded, deveined, and finely chopped (Wear plastic gloves when handling.)

½ bunch fresh cilantro, chopped

2 tomatoes, seeded and chopped

Juice of 4 limes

Kosher or sea salt

Cut the avocados lengthwise and remove the pits. Scoop out the flesh, place it in a bowl, and mash until chunky. Add the onion, jalapeños, cilantro, tomatoes, lime juice, and salt to taste. Mix well.

For best flavor, serve immediately. If storing, wrap the bowl tightly with plastic wrap or put the guacamole in an airtight container to prevent oxidation. Dip sliced veggies or approved crackers in it, or use it as a spread for burgers, chicken, or fish.

Makes 10 servings (4 cups)

Mediterranean Salad

2 cups dark leafy lettuce

¼ cup chopped cucumber

¼ cup chopped red bell pepper

½ small avocado, sliced

8 kalamata olives

1 ounce crumbled feta cheese

1 teaspoon olive oil

Juice of 1 lemon or lime

Cover your plate or storage container with the lettuce and top with the cucumber, pepper, avocado, olives, and cheese. Toss with the olive oil and lemon juice just before serving.

Makes 1 serving

Tomato and Mozzarella Salad

2 medium tomatoes, cut into wedges

2 ounces fresh mozzarella cheese, sliced

½ small avocado, sliced

1 tablespoon chopped fresh basil

2 tablespoons extra virgin olive oil

½ tablespoon balsamic vinegar

Salt and pepper

Combine the tomatoes, cheese, avocado, and basil in a small bowl. Drizzle the olive oil and vinegar on top. Season with salt and pepper. Serve as a snack or side dish. To turn into a lunchtime meal, serve over a bed of greens.

Makes 2 servings

Mashed Cauliflower

1 pound frozen cauliflower florets

2 tablespoons heavy cream

3 tablespoons unsalted butter, softened

Cayenne pepper or paprika

Microwave the cauliflower according to the package instructions, until very soft. Remove and drain off excess water. Mash the cauliflower with a wooden spoon or fork to squeeze out excess water, and drain. Place the cauliflower, cream, and butter in a food processor. Blend until creamy. Add cayenne pepper or paprika to taste.

Makes 3 servings

Garlicy Steamed Vegetables

1 tablespoon chopped leeks
3 cloves garlic, diced
1 tablespoon chopped chives
Pinch each of sea or kosher salt and pepper
2 cups chopped broccoli or cauliflower

Place the leeks, half of the garlic, chives, salt, and pepper in a medium pot. Fill halfway with water. Bring to a boil over high heat. Reduce the heat to low, cover, and cook for 7 to 10 minutes, or until the water takes on the aroma of the herbs. Place a steaming rack or bamboo steamer over the pot and place the broccoli and the remaining garlic in the basket. Cover and steam for 2 to 3 minutes, or until heated through.

Makes 1 serving

Cheesy Fruit

1 apple or pear
2 slices any cheese

Slice the apple into 8 thin strips. Top each strip with a bit of cheese. Put on a microwave-safe plate. Microwave for 20 seconds, or until the cheese melts.

Makes 2 servings

Baked Cheese

You can eat this snack alone or dipped in guacamole. It's a great option for people who crave crunchy snacks such as chips.

4 ounces any cheese

Preheat the oven to 350°F. Slice the cheese into 4 thin slices. Place the cheese slices on a baking sheet. Bake for 6 to 8 minutes, until the cheese melts and becomes brown on the edges.

Makes 1 serving

Avocado with Cheese

½ **avocado, pitted**
2 **tablespoons ricotta cheese**
Cayenne pepper or cumin (optional)

Fill the middle of the avocado with the ricotta cheese. Sprinkle the cayenne pepper on top (if using) and serve.

Makes 1 serving

Steak Fajitas

1 pound skirt steak

Sea or kosher salt and pepper

4 tablespoons unsalted butter

1 medium onion, sliced

1 clove garlic, chopped

1½ red, yellow, or green bell peppers, sliced

1 jalapeño chile pepper, chopped (Wear plastic gloves when handling.)

2 teaspoons chili powder or cayenne pepper

2 teaspoons ground cumin

2 to 4 tablespoons fresh tomato salsa

1 tablespoon Guacamole (page 232)

Chopped cilantro (optional)

Dash of hot sauce (optional)

Preheat the broiler. Season the steak with salt and pepper on both sides. In a broiler pan, broil for 4 minutes on each side (for rare to medium-rare). Remove from the broiler and let stand for a few minutes to cool. Slice into strips.

Heat a large skillet over high heat for 1 minute. Reduce the heat to medium and add 2 tablespoons of the butter. Rotate the skillet to evenly coat it with melted butter. Add the onion. Cook, stirring frequently, until the onion is soft and translucent, 2 to 3 minutes. If the liquid evaporates, add 2 tablespoons water. Add the garlic, bell peppers, jalapeño, chili powder, cumin, the remaining 2 tablespoons of butter and salt and papper to taste. Mix until completely coated, stirring frequently. Add water as needed. Once the peppers have softened, 2 to 3 minutes, add the sliced steak. Combine thoroughly.

Remove from the skillet and top with the salsa, guacamole, cilantro (if using), and hot sauce (if using).

Tip: If you would like the steak cooked a little more, just cover the plate after removing it from the oven. The meat will continue to cook.

Makes 4 servings

Meatballs Florentine

2¼ cups tomato sauce

1 bag (6 ounces) baby spinach

20 meatballs (1½ ounces each), cooked

¼ cup shredded mozzarella cheese

Place the sauce and spinach in a deep skillet. Cover and heat over medium-low heat, stirring occasionally, until the spinach wilts, 5 to 7 minutes. Add the meatballs and cook until they have warmed through, about 20 minutes. Sprinkle the cheese over the meatballs. Remove from the heat and let stand, covered, until the cheese melts, 3 to 5 minutes.

Makes 5 servings

Salmon on a "Bagel"

¼ beefsteak tomato, sliced into 2 thick slices

1 tablespoon cream cheese

¼ medium onion, thickly sliced

3 ounces smoked salmon

Place the tomato slices on a plate. Spread the cream cheese over each tomato and top with the onion and smoked salmon.

Makes 1 serving

Salmon with Mediterranean Salsa

Salsa

   1 cup chopped grape tomatoes
  10 kalamata olives, pitted and chopped
  ½ cup chopped red onion
  ½ large cucumber, peeled and chopped
  1½ tablespoons olive oil
   1 teaspoon red wine vinegar
     Pinch of dried basil
     Pinch of dried marjoram
     Pinch of dried oregano
     Pinch each of sea or kosher salt and pepper

To make the salsa: Place all of the ingredients in a bowl and stir to combine.

Salmon

   4 wild salmon fillets, 6 ounces each, deboned and skinned
     Sea salt and pepper
   1 tablespoon unsalted butter

To make the salmon: Season the salmon with salt and pepper on both sides. Set aside.

Melt the butter in a skillet over medium-high heat. Rotate the skillet to evenly coat it with butter. Add the salmon fillets. Cook for 2 to 3 minutes on each side (for medium-rare) or longer for desired doneness.

Divide the salsa among 4 plates and top with the salmon fillets.

Makes 4 servings

Tuna Melt

　1　can or package (6 to 7 ounces) tuna, drained
　1　rib celery, finely chopped
　2　tablespoons diced cucumber
　2　tablespoons diced onion
　1　tablespoon mayonnaise
　1　yellow bell pepper, halved and seeded
　1　slice any cheese

Preheat the oven to 400°F.

In a small bowl, combine the tuna, celery, cucumber, onion, and mayonnaise. Stuff the tuna mixture inside the bell pepper halves. Place the peppers on a baking sheet and top with the slice of cheese. Bake until the cheese melts, 3 to 5 minutes.

Makes 1 serving

Mexican Chicken Stir-Fry

2 tablespoons coconut oil

2 pounds boneless, skinless chicken breasts, chopped into bite-size pieces

2 cloves garlic, mashed

1 cup sliced onion

1 cup broccoli florets

1 cup sliced yellow bell pepper

⅔ cup salsa

Heat the oil in a wok or large skillet over medium-high heat. Add the chicken and garlic. Cook, stirring frequently, for 12 minutes, or until the chicken cooks through. Add the onion, broccoli, and pepper. Cover and cook for 6 to 8 minutes, or until the vegetables are crisp-tender. Remove from the heat. Add the salsa and combine thoroughly.

Serving suggestion: Top with Guacamole (page 232) and 2 to 3 tablespoons of chopped cilantro.

Makes 4 servings

Curry Chicken

1 pound boneless, skinless chicken breasts
Curry powder

Preheat the oven to 375°F.

Thoroughly season the chicken with curry powder to taste. Bake for 30 to 40 minutes, or until the internal temperature reads 165°F on an instant-read thermometer.

Makes 2 servings

Turkey Soup

3 cups chicken broth

1 package (10 ounces) frozen vegetables of your choice

7 ounces boneless, skinless turkey breast, cooked and cubed

Heat the broth in a saucepan over medium–high heat. Add the vegetables and cook until they warm though, 5 to 10 minutes. Add the turkey, heat through, and serve.

Makes 2 servings

LEVEL 2 RECIPES

The following recipes contain more starch and carbohydrate foods than you can eat on Level 1. Use them for Level 2 only.

Ice Cream Float

1 tablespoon unsweetened almond milk

⅓ cup zero-carb seltzer

½ cup natural vanilla ice cream

Pour the almond milk into an 8-ounce glass. Add the seltzer until the glass is ⅓ full. Stir gently. Add the ice cream and the remaining seltzer until the glass is full.

Makes 1 serving

Red Pepper Hummus

1 can (15.5 ounces) chickpeas, drained
(Reserve 2 tablespoons liquid.)

¼ cup organic sesame tahini

Juice of ½ lemon

1 clove garlic

2 whole roasted red bell peppers, skins removed

1 teaspoon kosher salt

1 teaspoon cracked ground pepper

¼ cup olive oil

2 tablespoons water

In a food processor, combine the chickpeas, reserved chickpea liquid, tahini, lemon juice, garlic, peppers, salt and pepper to taste, olive oil, and water. Blend until smooth. Refrigerate and serve with sliced vegetables.

Makes 8 servings (2 cups)

"Veggie" Burger

- 2 tablespoons coconut oil
- 1 medium onion, finely chopped
- 1 cup finely chopped mushrooms (Wild mushrooms are best.)
- 1 small zucchini, shredded
- 1 pound ground beef (90% lean will hold together better)
- 1 clove garlic, crushed
- 1 egg
- ¼ cup rolled oats
- ½ tablespoon paprika
- ¼ teaspoon celery seed
- ¼ teaspoon ground pepper
- 1 teaspoon salt

Place a skillet over medium heat. Add 1 tablespoon of the oil and the onion. Sauté until the onion is translucent, 3 to 4 minutes. Remove the onion and set aside. Place the mushrooms in the pan and sauté until they give up their water, about 5 minutes. When the majority of the water has reduced, place the onion back in the pan along with the zucchini. Sauté until the zucchini is just tender.

In a medium bowl, combine the beef, garlic, egg, oats, paprika, celery seed, pepper, and salt. Stir in the sautéed vegetables and form into 8 patties just smaller than your palm. Place the skillet back over medium heat. Add the remaining 1 tablespoon of oil, then add the burgers. Cook for 15 minutes or until desired doneness, flipping only once.

Makes 8 servings

Meatballs Florentine with Whole Grain Pasta

　3　cups tomato sauce

　1　bag (6 ounces) baby spinach

20　meatballs (1½ ounces each), cooked

　¼　cup shredded mozzarella cheese

1½　cups whole grain pasta, cooked according to package
　　 directions

Put the sauce and spinach in a deep skillet, cover, and place over medium-low heat. Stir occasionally until the spinach wilts, 5 to 7 minutes. Add the meatballs and cook until they have warmed through, about 20 minutes. Sprinkle the cheese over the meatballs. Remove from the heat and let stand, covered, until the cheese melts, 3 to 5 minutes. Serve over the pasta.

Makes 5 servings

Mexican Meatloaf

1 tablespoon grapeseed oil

1 large onion, finely chopped

2 cloves garlic, smashed

1 bunch spinach or other dark leafy green, chopped

1 can (16 ounces) black beans, rinsed and drained

1 teaspoon ground cumin

1 teaspoon ground ancho chile pepper

1 teaspoon salt

¼ teaspoon ground black pepper

1 teaspoon Mexican oregano

1 tablespoon chopped fresh cilantro

2 tablespoons mild salsa

1 tablespoon olive oil

1 pound 85% lean ground beef

1 egg

Salsa or Guacamole (see page 232) for serving (optional)

Preheat the oven to 350°F.

Place a large skillet over medium-high heat. Add the grapeseed oil and chopped onion. Sauté until the onion is translucent, 2 to 3 minutes. Add the garlic; cook for 30 seconds longer. Add the greens; cook until wilted and most of the water has boiled off. Remove from the heat.

Place the beans in a medium saucepan over medium-low heat. Add the cumin, chile pepper, salt, black pepper, oregano, cilantro, and salsa. Cook for 20 minutes, stirring occasionally. Near the end of the cooking time, stir in the olive oil. The beans should start to break up.

Place the beef in a medium bowl. Mix in the egg, greens, and cooked beans. Place the meat mixture in a standard-size loaf pan. Cover with foil. Bake in the oven for 1 to 1½ hours, or until an instant-read thermometer inserted in the center of the loaf registers 175°F.

Remove from the oven. Cool for 10 minutes. Remove from the loaf pan, slice, and serve. Top with salsa or guacamole (if using) for extra flavor.

Makes 6 servings

Ambrosia

½ cup cottage cheese

2 tablespoons Greek 2% yogurt

1 tablespoon nuts

1 tablespoon flaxseed

½ small tangerine, sliced and seeded

¼ banana, sliced

Dash of cinnamon (optional)

Combine the cottage cheese, yogurt, nuts, flaxseed, tangerine, banana, and cinnamon (if using) in a bowl and serve.

Makes 2 servings

Power Oatmeal

¼ cup steel cut oats

1 tablespoon crushed pecans

1 tablespoon flaxseed

½ tablespoon cinnamon

1 teaspoon heavy cream

1 teaspoon vanilla extract

Cook the oats according to the package instructions. Combine the cooked oats, pecans, flaxseed, cinnamon, cream, and vanilla extract in a bowl and serve.

Makes 1 serving

Hungry Man's Salad

    3 cups dark leafy lettuce
    2 hard-boiled eggs, sliced
    ½ small avocado, sliced
    ¼ cup chopped cucumber
    ¼ cup chopped red bell pepper
    ¼ cup chickpeas
    ¼ cup sliced grilled portobello mushroom
    3 ounces cooked chicken or turkey
    2 ounces goat cheese
    1 tablespoon pumpkin seeds

On a large plate or in a storage container, combine the lettuce, eggs, avocado, cucumber, pepper, chickpeas, mushroom, chicken or turkey, cheese, and pumpkin seeds.

Makes 2 servings, or 1 serving for a hungry man

Body Mass Index Table

Category	Normal						Overweight					Obese										Extreme Obesity													
BMI	19	20	21	22	23	24	25	26	27	28	29	30	31	32	33	34	35	36	37	38	39	40	41	42	43	44	45	46	47	48	49	50	51	52	53	54
Height (inches)																	Body Weight (pounds)																			
58	91	96	100	105	110	115	119	124	129	134	138	143	148	153	158	162	167	172	177	181	186	191	196	201	205	210	215	220	224	229	234	239	244	248	253	258
59	94	99	104	109	114	119	124	128	133	138	143	148	153	158	163	168	173	178	183	188	193	198	203	208	212	217	222	227	232	237	242	247	252	257	262	267
60	97	102	107	112	118	123	128	133	138	143	148	153	158	163	168	174	179	184	189	194	199	204	209	215	220	225	230	235	240	245	250	255	261	266	271	276
61	100	106	111	116	122	127	132	137	143	148	153	158	164	169	174	180	185	190	195	201	206	211	217	222	227	232	238	243	248	254	259	264	269	275	280	285
62	104	109	115	120	126	131	136	142	147	153	158	164	169	175	180	186	191	196	202	207	213	218	224	229	235	240	246	251	256	262	267	273	278	284	289	295
63	107	113	118	124	130	135	141	146	152	158	163	169	175	180	186	191	197	203	208	214	220	225	231	237	242	248	254	259	265	270	278	282	287	293	299	304
64	110	116	122	128	134	140	145	151	157	163	169	174	180	186	192	197	204	209	215	221	227	232	238	244	250	256	262	267	273	279	285	291	296	302	308	314
65	114	120	126	132	138	144	150	156	162	168	174	180	186	192	198	204	210	216	222	228	234	240	246	252	258	264	270	276	282	288	294	300	306	312	318	324
66	118	124	130	136	142	148	155	161	167	173	179	186	192	198	204	210	216	223	229	235	241	247	253	260	266	272	278	284	291	297	303	309	315	322	328	334
67	121	127	134	140	146	153	159	166	172	178	185	191	198	204	211	217	223	230	236	242	249	255	261	268	274	280	287	293	299	306	312	319	325	331	338	344
68	125	131	138	144	151	158	164	171	177	184	190	197	203	210	216	223	230	236	243	249	256	262	269	276	282	289	295	302	308	315	322	328	335	341	348	354
69	128	135	142	149	155	162	169	176	182	189	196	203	209	216	223	230	236	243	250	257	263	270	277	284	291	297	304	311	318	324	331	338	345	351	358	365
70	132	139	146	153	160	167	174	181	188	195	202	209	216	222	229	236	243	250	257	264	271	278	285	292	299	306	313	320	327	334	341	348	355	362	369	376
71	136	143	150	157	165	172	179	186	193	200	208	215	222	229	236	243	250	257	265	272	279	286	293	301	308	315	322	329	338	343	351	358	365	372	379	386
72	140	147	154	162	169	177	184	191	199	206	213	221	228	235	242	250	258	265	272	279	287	294	302	309	316	324	331	338	346	353	361	368	375	383	390	397
73	144	151	159	166	174	182	189	197	204	212	219	227	235	242	250	257	265	272	280	288	295	302	310	318	325	333	340	348	355	363	371	378	386	393	401	408
74	148	155	163	171	179	186	194	202	210	218	225	233	241	249	256	264	272	280	287	295	303	311	319	326	334	342	350	358	365	373	381	389	396	404	412	420
75	152	160	168	176	184	192	200	208	216	224	232	240	248	256	264	272	279	287	295	303	311	319	327	335	343	351	359	367	375	383	391	399	407	415	423	431
76	156	164	172	180	189	197	205	213	221	230	238	246	254	263	271	279	287	295	304	312	320	328	336	344	353	361	369	377	385	394	402	410	418	426	435	443

Source: Adapted from Clinical Guidelines on the Identification, Evaluation, and Treatment of Overweight and Obesity in Adults: The Evidence Report.

BIBLIOGRAPHY

CHAPTER 2

Basciano, H., L. Federico, and K. Adeli. "Fructose, Insulin Resistance, and Metabolic Dyslipidemia." *Nutrition and Metabolism* 2, no. 1 (February 2005): 5.

Beyer, P. L., E. M. Caviar, and R. W. McCallum. "Fructose Intake at Current Levels in the United States May Cause Gastrointestinal Distress in Normal Adults." *Journal of the American Dietetic Association* 105, no. 10 (October 2005): 1559–66.

Bray, G. A., S. J. Nielsen, and B. M. Popkin. "Consumption of High-Fructose Corn Syrup in Beverages May Play a Role in the Epidemic of Obesity." *American Journal of Clinical Nutrition* 79, no. 4 (April 2004): 537–43.

Chavarro, J. E., T. L. Toth, S. M. Sadio, and R. Hauser. "Soy Food and Isoflavone Intake in Relation to Semen Quality Parameters among Men from an Infertility Clinic." *Human Reproduction* (July 23, 2008), doi: 10.1093/humrep/den243.

Elliott, S. S., N. L. Keim, J. S. Stern, K. Teff, and P. J. Havel. "Fructose, Weight Gain, and the Insulin Resistance Syndrome." *American Journal of Clinical Nutrition* 76, no. 5 (November 2002): 911–22.

Fields, S. "The Fat of the Land: Do Agricultural Subsidies Foster Poor Health?" *Environmental Health Perspectives* 112, no. 14 (October 2004): A820–3.

Gao, X., L. Qi, N. Qiao, H. K. Choi, G. Curhan, K. L. Tucker, and A. Ascherio. "Intake of Added Sugar and Sugar-Sweetened Drink and Serum Uric Acid Concentration in US Men and Women." *Hypertension* 50, no. 2 (August 2007): 306–12.

Ishizuki, Y., et al. "The Effects on the Thyroid Gland of Soybeans Administered Experimentally in Healthy Subjects." *Nippon Naibunpi Gakkai Zasshi* 67, no. 5 (1991): 622–29.

Kumar, K., S. C. Gupta, S. K. Baidoo, Y. Chander, and C. J. Rosen. "Antibiotic Uptake by Plants from Soil Fertilized with Animal Manure." *Journal of Environmental Quality* 34, no. 6 (October 12, 2005): 2082–85.

Lingelbach, L. B., and R. B. McDonald. "Description of the Long-Term Lipogenic Effects of Dietary Carbohydrates in Male Fischer 344 Rats." *Journal of Nutrition* 130, no. 12 (December 2000): 3077–84.

Mazer, N. A. "Interaction of Estrogen Therapy and Thyroid Hormone Replacement in Postmenopausal Women." *Thyroid* 14, Suppl no. 1 (2004): S27–34.

Messina, M., C. Nagata, and A. H. Wu. "Estimated Asian Adult Soy Protein and Isoflavone Intakes." *Nutrition and Cancer* 55, no. 1 (2006): 1–12.

Messina, M., and G. Redmond. "Effects of Soy Protein and Soybean Isoflavones on Thyroid Function in Healthy Adults and Hypothyroid Patients: A Review of the Relevant Literature." *Thyroid* 16, no. 3 (March 2006): 249–58.

Milerová, J., J. Cerovská, V. Zamrazil, R. Bílek, O. Lapčík, and R. Hampl. "Actual Levels of Soy Phytoestrogens in Children Correlate with Thyroid Laboratory Parameters." *Clinical Chemistry and Laboratory Medicine* 44, no. 2 (2006): 171–74.

Nakagawa, T., H. Hu, S. Zharikov, K. R. Tuttle, R. A. Short, O. Glushakova, X. Ouyang, et al. "A Causal Role for Uric Acid in Fructose-Induced Metabolic Syndrome." *American Journal of Physiology—Renal Physiology* 290, no. 3 (March 2006): F625–31.

USDA Database for Added Sugars Content of Selected Foods Release 1, February 2006.

Yoshida, M., N. M. McKeown, G. Rogers, J. B. Meigs, E. Saltzman, R. D'Agostino, and P. F. Jacques. "Surrogate Markers of Insulin Resistance Are Associated with Consumption of Sugar-Sweetened Drinks and Fruit Juice in Older-Aged Adults." *Journal of Nutrition* 137 (September 2007): 2121–27.

Ziegler, E. E. "Growth of Breast-Fed and Formula-Fed Infants." Nestlé Nutrition Workshop Series Pediatric Program, no. 58 (2006): 51–9.

CHAPTER 3

Anderson, J. W., E. C. Konz, and D. J. A. Jenkins. "Health Advantages and Disadvantages of Weight-Reducing Diets: A Computer Analysis and Critical Review." *Journal of the American College of Nutrition* 19 (2000): 578–90.

Dhingra, R., L. Sullivan, P. F. Jacques, T. J. Wang, C. S. Fox, J. B. Meigs, R. B. D'Agostino, J. M. Gaziano, and R. S. Vasan. "Soft Drink Consumption and Risk of Developing Cardiometabolic Risk Factors and the Metabolic Syndrome in Middle-Aged Adults in the Community." *Circulation* 116, no. 5 (July 2007): 480–88.

Ding, H., Y. W. Chin, A. D. Kinghorn, and S. M. D'Ambrosio. "Chemopreventive Characteristics of Avocado Fruit." *Seminars in Cancer Biology* 17, no. 5 (October 2007): 386–94.

Field, A. E., W. C. Willett, L. Lissner, and G. A. Colditz. "Dietary Fat and Weight Gain among Women in the Nurses' Health Study." *Obesity* 15, no. 4 (April 2007): 967–76.

Gardner, C. D., A. Kiazand, S. Alhassan, S. Kim, R. S. Stafford, R. R. Balise, H. C. Kraemer, and A. C. King. "Comparison of the Atkins, Zone, Ornish, and LEARN Diets for Change in Weight and Related Risk Factors among Overweight Premenopausal Women: The A TO Z Weight Loss Study: A Randomized Trial." *Journal of the American Medical Association* 297, no. 9 (March 2007): 969–77.

Hayes, M., C. Miller, J. Ulbrecht, J. Mauger, L. Parker-Klees, M. Gutschall, D. Mitchell, H. Smiciklas-Wright, and M. Covasa. "A Carbohydrate-Restricted Diet Alters Gut Peptides and Adiposity Signals in Men and Women with Metabolic Syndrome." *Journal of Nutrition* 26, no. 137 (July 2007): 1944–50.

Ludwig, A. K., J. M. Weiss, S. Tauchert, T. Dietze, S. Rudolf, K. Diedrich, A. Peters, and K. M. Oltmanns. "Influence of Hypo- and Hyperglycemia on Plasma Leptin Concentrations in Healthy Women and in Women with Polycystic Ovary Syndrome." *Human Reproduction* 22, no. 6 (June 2007): 1555–61.

Morgan, L., B. Griffin, D. Millward, A. Delooy, K. Fox, S. Baic, M. Bonham, et al. "Comparison of the Effects of Four Commercially Available Weight-Loss Programs on Lipid-Based Cardiovascular Risk Factors." *Public Health Nutrition* 23 (July 2008): 1–9.

Pereira, M. A., J. Swain, A. B. Goldfine, N. Rifai, and D. S. Ludwig. "Effects of a Low-Glycemic Load Diet on Resting Energy Expenditure and Heart Disease Risk Factors during Weight Loss." *Journal of the American Medical Association* 292, no. 20 (November 2004): 2482–90.

Shai, I., D. Schwarzfuchs, Y. Henkin, D. R. Shahar, S. Witkow, I. Greenberg, R. Golan, et al. Dietary Intervention Randomized Controlled Trial (DIRECT) Group. "Weight Loss with a Low-Carbohydrate, Mediterranean, or Low-Fat Diet." *New England Journal of Medicine* 359, no. 3 (July 2008): 229–41.

Taylor, E., E. Missik, R. Hurley, S. Hudak, and E. Logue. "Obesity Treatment: Broadening Our Perspective." *American Journal of Health Behavior* 28, no. 3 (2004): 242–49.

Welle, S., U. Lilavivat, and R. G. Campbell. "Thermic Effect of Feeding in Man: Increased Plasma Norepinephrine Levels Following Glucose but Not Protein or Fat Consumption." *Metabolism: Clinical and Experimental* 30, no. 10 (October 1981): 953–958.

Yoshida, M., N. M. McKeown, G. Rogers, J. B. Meigs, E. Saltzman, R. D'Agostino, and P. F. Jacques. "Surrogate Markers of Insulin Resistance Are Associated with Consumption of Sugar-Sweetened Drinks and Fruit Juice in Older-Aged Adults." *Journal of Nutrition* 137 (September 2007): 2121–27.

CHAPTER 4

Bray, G. A., M. Most, J. Rood, S. Redmann, and S. R. Smith. "Hormonal Responses to a Fast-Food Meal Compared with Nutritionally Comparable Meals of Different Composition." *Annals of Nutrition and Metabolism* 51, no. 2 (2007): 163–71.

Castelli, W. "Framingham Heart Study: Saturated Fat and Cholesterol not Linked to Heart Disease or Weight Gain." *Archives of Internal Medicine* 152, no. 7 (July 1992): 1371–72.

Chan, J. M., M. J. Stampfer, J. Ma, P. H. Gann, J. M. Gaziano, and E. L. Giovannucci. "Dairy Products, Calcium, and Prostate Cancer Risk in the Physicians' Health Study." *American Journal of Clinical Nutrition* 74, no. 4 (October 2001): 549–54.

Chavarro, J. E., J. W. Rich-Edwards, B. A. Rosner, and W. C. Willett. "Dietary Fatty Acid Intakes and the Risk of Ovulatory Infertility." *American Journal of Clinical Nutrition* 85, no. 1 (January 2007): 231–37.

DeFronzo, R., and E. Ferrannini. "Insulin Resistance—A Multifaceted Syndrome Responsible for NIDDM, Obesity, Hypertension, Dyslipidemia, and Atherosclerotic Cardiovascular Disease." *Diabetes Care* 4, no. 3 (1991): 173–94.

Denke, M. A. "Dietary Fats, Fatty Acids, and Their Effects on Lipoproteins." *Current Atherosclerosis Reports* 8, no. 6 (November 2006): 466–71.

Dreon, D. M., H. A. Fernstrom, H. Campos, P. Blanche, P. T. Williams, and R. M. Krauss. "Change in Dietary Saturated Fat Intake Is Correlated with Change in Mass of Large Low-Density-Lipoprotein Particles in Men." *American Journal of Clinical Nutrition* 67, no. 5 (May 1998): 828–36.

Dreon, D. M., H. A. Fernstrom, P. T. Williams, and R. M. Krauss. "LDL Subclass Patterns and Lipoprotein Response to a Low-Fat, High-Carbohydrate Diet in Women." *Arteriosclerosis, Thrombosis, and Vascular Biology* 17, no. 4 (April 1997): 707–14.

Dreon, D. M., H. A. Fernstrom, P. T. Williams, and R. M. Krauss. "Reduced LDL Particle Size in Children Consuming a Very Low-Fat Diet Is Related to Parental LDL-Subclass Patterns." *American Journal of Clinical Nutrition* 71, no. 6 (June 2000): 1611–16.

Dreon, D. M., H. A. Fernstrom, P. T. Williams, and R. M. Krauss. "A Very Low-Fat Diet Is Not Associated with Improved Lipoprotein Profiles in Men with a Predominance of Large, Low-Density Lipoproteins." *American Journal of Clinical Nutrition* 69, no. 3 (March 1999): 411–18.

Folaron, I., and T. Sauerwein. "Hyperinsulinemic Hypoglycemia Following Roux-en-Y Gastric Bypass Surgery." *Practical Diabetology* 3, no. 11(March 2006): 10–18.

Gapstur, S. M., and S. Khan. "Fat, Fruits, Vegetables, and Breast Cancer Survivorship." *Journal of the American Medical Association* 298, no. 3 (July 2007): 289–98, 335–36.

Genkinger, J. M., D. J. Hunter, D. Spiegelman, K. E. Anderson, A. Arslan, W. L. Beeson, J. E. Buring, et al. "Dairy Products and Ovarian Cancer: A Pooled Analysis of 12 Cohort Studies." *Cancer Epidemiology Biomarkers & Prevention* 15, no. 2 (February 2006): 364–72.

Genkinger, J. M., D. J. Hunter, D. Spiegelman, K. E. Anderson, W. L. Beeson, J. E. Buring, G. A. Colditz, et al. "A Pooled Analysis of 12 Cohort Studies of Dietary Fat, Cholesterol, and Egg Intake and Ovarian Cancer." *Cancer Causes & Control* 17, no. 3 (April 2006): 273–85.

Gerster, H. "Can Adults Adequately Convert Alpha-Linolenic Acid (18:3n-3) to Eicosapentaenoic Acid (20:5n-3) and Docosahexaenoic Acid (22:6n-3)?" *International Journal for Vitamin and Nutrition Research* 68, no. 3 (1998): 159–73.

Halton, T. L., W. C. Willett, S. Liu, J. E. Manson, C. M. Albert, K. Rexrode, and F. B. Hu. "Low-Carbohydrate-Diet Score and the Risk of Coronary Heart Disease in Women." *New England Journal of Medicine* 355, no. 19 (November 2006): 1991–2002.

Howard, B., L. Van Horn, J. Hsia, et al. "Low-Fat Dietary Pattern and Risk of Cardiovascular Disease." *Journal of the American Medical Association* 295, no. 6 (February 2006): 655–666.

Kim, E. H., W. C. Willett, G. A Colditz, S. E. Hankinson, M. J. Stampfer, D. J. Hunter, B. Rosner, and M. D. Holmes. "Dietary Fat and Risk of Postmenopausal Breast Cancer in a 20-Year Follow-Up." *American Journal of Epidemiology* 164, no. 10 (November 2006): 990–97.

Knopp, R., and B. Retzlaff. "Saturated Fat Prevents Coronary Artery Disease? An American Paradox." *American Journal of Clinical Nutrition* 80, no. 5 (November 2004): 1102–103.

Koh-Banerjee, P., N. F. Chu, D. Spiegelman, B. Rosner, G. Colditz, W. Willett, and E. Rimm. "Prospective Study of the Association of

Changes in Dietary Intake, Physical Activity, Alcohol Consumption, and Smoking with 9-Year Gain in Waist Circumference among 16,587 US Men." *American Journal of Clinical Nutrition* 78, no. 4 (October 2003): 719–27.

Krauss, R. M., and D. M. Dreon. "Low-Density-Lipoprotein Subclasses and Response to a Low-Fat Diet in Healthy Men." *American Journal of Clinical Nutrition* 62, no. 2 (August 1995): 478S–87S.

Lichtenstein, A. "Dietary Fat, Carbohydrate, and Protein: Effects on Plasma Lipoprotein Profiles, Fat, Carbohydrate, and Protein Plasma Lipids." *Journal of Lipid Research* (August 2007): 1661–1667

Lieberman, D. A., S. Prindiville, D. G. Weiss, and W. Willett. VA Cooperative Study Group 380. "Risk Factors for Advanced Colonic Neoplasia and Hyperplastic Polyps in Asymptomatic Individuals." *Journal of the American Medical Association* 290, no. 22 (December 2003): 2959–67.

Maki, K., T. Rains, V. Kaden, K. Raneri, and M. Davidson. "Effects of a Reduced-Glycemic-Load Diet on Body Weight, Body Composition, and Cardiovascular Disease Risk Markers in Overweight and Obese Adults." *American Journal of Clinical Nutrition* 85, no. 3 (March 2007): 724–34.

Michaud, D. S., H. G. Skinner, K. Wu, F. Hu, E. Giovannucci, W. C. Willett, G. A. Colditz, and C. S. Fuchs. "Dietary Patterns and Pancreatic Cancer Risk in Men and Women." *Journal of the National Cancer Institute* 97, no. 7 (April 2005): 518–24.

Moretti, L., and T. Canada. "A Randomized Study Comparing the Effects of a Low-Carbohydrate Diet and a Conventional Diet on Lipoprotein Subfractions and C-reactive Protein Levels in Patients with Severe Obesity." *American Journal of Clinical Nutrition* 83, no. 4 (April 2006): 760–66.

Morgan, L., B. Griffin, D. Millward, A. Delooy, K. Fox, S. Baic, M. Bonham, et al. "Comparison of the Effects of Four Commercially Available Weight-Loss Programs on Lipid-Based Cardiovascular Risk Factors." *Public Health Nutrition* (July 2008): 1–9.

Mozaffarian, D., E. Rimm, and D. Herrington. "Dietary Fats, Carbohy-drate, and Progression of Coronary Atherosclerosis in Postmenopausal Women." *American Journal of Clinical Nutrition* 80, no. 5 (November 2004): 1175–84.

Nazarewicz, R. R., W. Ziolkowski, P. S. Vaccaro, and P. Ghafourifar. "Effect of Short-Term Ketogenic Diet on Redox Status of Human Blood." *Rejuvenation Research* 10, no. 4 (July 2007): 335–440.

Oh, K., F. B. Hu, J. E. Manson, M. J. Stampfer, and W. C. Willett. "Dietary Fat Intake and Risk of Coronary Heart Disease in Women:

20 Years of Follow-up of the Nurses' Health Study." *American Journal of Epidemiology* 161, no. 7 (April 2005): 672–79.

Reaven, G. "Role of Insulin Resistance in Human Disease." *Diabetes* 37 (1988): 1595–1607.

Reaven, G. "Syndrome X." *Clinical Diabetes* 3–4 (1994): 32–52.

Romieu, I., E. Lazcano-Ponce, L. M. Sanchez-Zamorano, W. Willett, and M. Hernandez-Avila. "Carbohydrates and the Risk of Breast Cancer among Mexican Women." *Cancer Epidemiology, Biomarkers & Prevention* 13, no. 8 (August 2004): 1283–89.

Shai I., D. Schwarzfuchs, Y. Henkin, D. R. Shahar, S. Witkow, I. Greenberg, and R. Golan. Dietary Intervention Randomized Controlled Trial (DIRECT) Group. "Weight Loss with a Low-Carbohydrate, Mediterranean, or Low-Fat Diet." *New England Journal of Medicine* 359, no. 3 (July 2008): 229–41.

Shin, M. J., P. J. Blanche, R. S. Rawlings, H. S. Fernstrom, and R. M. Krauss. "Increased Plasma Concentrations of Lipoprotein(a) During a Low-Fat, High-Carbohydrate Diet Are Associated with Increased Plasma Concentrations of Apolipoprotein C-III Bound to Apolipoprotein B-Containing Lipoproteins." *American Journal of Clinical Nutrition* 85, no. 6 (June 2007): 1527–32.

Smith, R. N., N. J. Mann, A. Braue, H. Mäkeläinen, and G. A. Varigos. "The Effect of a High-Protein, Low-Glycemic-Load Diet versus a Conventional, High-Glycemic-Load Diet on Biochemical Parameters Associated with Acne Vulgaris: A Randomized, Investigator-Masked, Controlled Trial." *Journal of the American Academy of Dermatology* 57, no. 2 (August 2007): 247–56.

Smith, R. N., N. J. Mann, A. Braue, H. Mäkeläinen, and G. A. Varigos. "A Low-Glycemic-Load Diet Improves Symptoms in Acne Vulgaris Patients: A Randomized Controlled Trial." *American Journal of Clinical Nutrition* 86, no. 1 (July 2007): 107–15.

Sun, Q., J. Ma, H. Campos, S. E. Hankinson, J. E. Manson, M. J. Stampfer, K. M. Rexrode, W. C. Willett, and F. B. Hu. "A Prospective Study of Trans Fatty Acids in Erythrocytes and Risk of Coronary Heart Disease." *Circulation* 115, no. 14 (April 2007): 1858–65.

Zaloga, G. P., K. A. Harvey, W. Stillwell, and R. Siddiqui. "Trans Fatty Acids and Coronary Heart Disease." *Nutrition in Clinical Practice: Official Publication of the Society for Parenteral and Enteral Nutrition* 21, no. 5 (October 2006): 505–12.

Zavoroni, I., et al. "Risk Factors for Coronary Artery Disease in Healthy Persons with Hyperinsulinemia and Normal Glucose Tolerance." *New England Journal of Medicine* 320 (1989): 702–706.

CHAPTER 5

Green, M. W., N. A. Elliman, and M. J. Kretsch. "Weight Loss Strategies, Stress, and Cognitive Function: Supervised versus Unsupervised Dieting." *Psychoneuroendocrinology* 30, no. 9 (October 2005): 908–18.

CHAPTER 6

Amarasiri, W. A., and A. S. Dissanayake. "Coconut Fats." *Ceylon Medical Journal* 51, no. 2 (June 2006): 47–51.

Bizeau, M. E., and J. R. Hazel. "Dietary Fat Type Alters Glucose Metabolism in Isolated Rat Hepatocytes." *Journal of Nutritional Biochemistry* 10, no. 12 (December 1999): 709–15.

Lukashev, D., A. Ohta, and M. Sitkovsky. "Hypoxia-Dependent Anti-inflammatory Pathways in Protection of Cancerous Tissues." *Cancer Metastasis Reviews* 26, no. 2 (June 2007): 273–79.

Mahmud, A., and J. Feely. "Acute Effect of Caffeine on Arterial Stiffness and Aortic Pressure Waveform." *Hypertension* 38, no. 2 (August 2001): 227–31.

Nevin, K. G., and T. Rajamohan. "Beneficial Effects of Virgin Coconut Oil on Lipid Parameters and In Vitro LDL Oxidation." *Clinical Biochemisty* 37, no. 9 (September 2004): 830–35.

Sitkovsky, M. V., and A. Ohta. "The 'Danger' Sensors That STOP the Immune Response: The A2 Adenosine Receptors?" *Trends in Immunology* 26, no. 6 (June 2005): 299–304.

St-Onge, M. P., and A. Bosarge. "Weight-Loss Diet That Includes Consumption of Medium-Chain Triacylglycerol Oil Leads to a Greater Rate of Weight and Fat Mass Loss Than Does Olive Oil." *American Journal of Clinical Nutrition* 87, no. 3 (March 2008): 621–26.

Vlachopoulos, C., K. Hirata, and M. F. O'Rourke. "Effect of Caffeine on Aortic Elastic Properties and Wave Reflection." *Journal of Hypertension* 21, no. 3 (March 2003): 563–70.

Wannamethee, S. G., and A. G. Shaper. "Alcohol, Body Weight, and Weight Gain in Middle-Aged Men." *American Journal of Clinical Nutrition* 77, no. 5 (May 2003): 1312–17.

CHAPTER 9

Althuis, M. D., N. E. Jordan, E. A. Ludington, and J. T. Wittes. "Glucose and Insulin Responses to Dietary Chromium Supplements: A Meta-analysis." *American Journal of Clinical Nutrition* 761, no. 1 (2002): 148–55.

Anderson, R. A. "Cinnamon, Glucose Tolerance, and Diabetes." Washington, DC: USDA Agricultural Research Service, 2005.

Anderson, R. A. "Effects of Chromium on Body Composition and Weight Loss." *Nutrition Reviews* 56, no. 9 (1998): 266–70.

Autier, P., and S. Gandini. "Vitamin D Supplementation and Total Mortality: A Meta-analysis of Randomized Controlled Trials." *Archives of Internal Medicine* 167, no. 16 (2007): 1730–37.

Bertone-Johnson, E. R., S. E. Hankinson, A. Bendich, S. R. Johnson, W. C. Willett, and J. E. Manson. "Calcium and Vitamin D Intake and Risk of Incident Premenstrual Syndrome." *Archives of Internal Medicine* 165, no. 11 (June 2005): 1246–52.

Coggeshall, J. C., J. P. Heggers, M. C. Robson, and H. Baker. "Biotin Status and Plasma Glucose Levels in Diabetics." *Annals of the New York Academy of Science* 447 (1985): 389–92.

Colombo, V. E., F. Gerber, M. Bronhofer, and G. L. Floersheim. "Treatment of Brittle Fingernails and Onychoschizia with Biotin: Scanning Electron Microscopy." *Journal of the American Academy of Dermatology* 23, 6 pt. 1 (1990): 1127–32.

Costell, M., J. E. O'Connor, and S. Grisolia. "Age-Dependent Decrease of Carnitine Content in Muscle of Mice and Humans." *Biochemical and Biophysical Research Communications* 161, no. 3 (1989): 1135–43.

Cramer, D. W. "Lactase Persistence and Milk Consumption as Determinants of Ovarian Cancer Risk." *American Journal of Epidemiology* 130 (1989): 904–10.

Cramer, D. W., B. L. Harlow, W. C. Willett, et al. "Galactose Consumption and Metabolism in Relation to the Risk of Ovarian Cancer." *Lancet* 2 (1989): 66–71.

Cummings, N. K., A. P. James, and M. J. Soares. "The Acute Effects of Different Sources of Dietary Calcium on Postprandial Energy Metabolism." *British Journal of Nutrition* 96, no. 1 (July 2006): 138–44.

DiBaise, J. K., H. Zhang, M. D. Crowell, R. Krajmalnik-Brown, G. A. Decker, and B. E. Rittmann. "Gut Microbiota and Its Possible Relationship with Obesity." *Mayo Clinic Proceedings* 83, no. 4 (April 2008): 460–69.

Eagan, M. S., R. M. Lyle, C. W. Gunther, M. Peacock, and D. Teegarden. "Effect of 1-Year Dairy Product Intervention on Fat Mass in Young Women: 6-Month Follow-up." *Obesity* 14, no. 12 (December 2006): 2242–48.

Fletcher, R. H., and K. M. Fairfield. "Vitamins for Chronic Disease Prevention in Adults." *Journal of American Medical Association* 287, no. 23 (2002): 3127–29.

Floersheim, G. L. "Treatment of Brittle Fingernails with Biotin." *Zeitschrift für Hautkrankheiten* 64, no. 1 (1989): 41–48.

Giovannucci, E., E. B. Rimm, A. Wolk, et al. "Calcium and Fructose Intake in Relation to Risk of Prostate Cancer." *Cancer Research* 58 (1998): 442–47.

Grau, M. V., J. A. Baron, R. S. Sandler, R. W. Haile, M. L. Beach, T. R. Church, and D. Heber. "Vitamin D, Calcium Supplementation, and Colorectal Adenomas: Results of a Randomized Trial." *Journal of the National Cancer Institute* 95, no. 23 (December 2003): 1765–71.

Hagen, T. M., R. T. Ingersoll, C. M. Wehr, et al. "Acetyl-L-Carnitine Fed to Old Rats Partially Restores Mitochondrial Function and Ambulatory Activity." *Proceedings of the National Academy of Science* 95, no. 16 (1998): 9562–66.

Hagen, T. M., J. Liu, J. Lykkesfeldt, et al. "Feeding Acetyl-L-Carnitine and Lipoic Acid to Old Rats Significantly Improves Metabolic Function while Decreasing Oxidative Stress." *Proceedings of the National Academy of Science* 99, no. 4 (2002): 1870–75.

Heaney, R., K. Rafferty, M. Dowell, and J. Bierman. "Calcium Fortification Systems Differ in Bioavailability." *Journal of the American Dietetic Association* 105, no. 5 (May 2005): 807–809.

Hochman, L. G., R. K. Scher, and M. S. Meyerson. "Brittle Nails: Response to Daily Biotin Supplementation." *Cutaneous Medicine for the Practitioner* 51, no. 4 (1993): 303–305.

Khan, Alam, Mahpara Safdar, Mohammad Muzaffar, Ali Khan, Khan Nawaz Khattak and Richard A. Anderson, "Cinnamon Improves Glucose and Lipids of People with Type 2 Diabetes." *Diabetes Care* 26 (2003): 3215–18.

Kobla, H. V., and S. L. Volpe. "Chromium, Exercise, and Body Composition." *Critical Reviews in Food Science and Nutrition* 40, no. 4 (2000): 291–308.

Kovacs, E. M. R., and D. J. Mela. "Metabolically Active Functional Food Ingredients for Weight Control." *Obesity Reviews* 7 (2006): 59–78.

Kris-Etherton, P. M., W. S. Harris, and L. J. Appel. "Fish Consumption, Fish Oil, Omega-3 Fatty Acids, and Cardiovascular Disease." *Circulation* 106 (2002): 2747–2757.

Liu, J., E. Head, A. M. Gharib, et al. "Memory Loss in Old Rats Is Associated with Brain Mitochondrial Decay and RNA/DNA Oxidation: Partial Reversal by Feeding Acetyl-L-Carnitine and/or R-Alpha-Lipoic Acid." *Proceedings of the National Academy of Science* 99, no. 4 (2002): 2356–61.

Maebashi, M., Y. Makino, Y. Furukawa, K. Ohinata, S. Kimura, and T. Sato. "Therapeutic Evaluation of the Effect of Biotin on Hyperglycemia in Patients with Non-insulin-Dependent Diabetes Mellitus." *Journal of Clinical Biochemistry and Nutrition* 14 (1993): 211–18.

Mertz, W. "Chromium in Human Nutrition: A Review." *Journal of Nutrition* 123, no. 4 (1993): 626–33.

Negro, R., G. Greco, T. Mangieri, A. Pezzarossa, D. Dazzi, and H. Hassan. "The Influence of Selenium Supplementation on Postpartum Thyroid Status in Pregnant Women with Thyroid Peroxidase Autoantibodies." *Journal of Clinical Endocrinology and Metabolism* 92, no. 4 (April 2007): 1263–68.

Olivares, M., M. P. Díaz-Ropero, S. Sierra, F. Lara-Villoslada, J. Fonollá, M. Navas, J. M. Rodríguez, and J. Xaus. "Oral Intake of *Lactobacillus fermentum* CECT5716 Enhances the Effects of Influenza Vaccination." *Nutrition* 23, no. 3 (March 2007): 254–60.

Pittler, M. H., C. Stevinson, and E. Ernst. "Chromium Picolinate for Reducing Body Weight: Meta-analysis of Randomized Trials." *International Journal of Obesity and Related Metabolism Disorders* 27, no. 4 (2003): 522–29.

Romero-Navarro, G., G. Cabrera-Valladares, M. S. German, et al. "Biotin Regulation of Pancreatic Glucokinase and Insulin in Primary Cultured Rat Islets and in Biotin-Deficient Rats." *Endocrinology* 140, no. 10 (1999): 4595–600.

Roongpisuthipong, C., R. Kantawan, and W. Roongpisuthipong. "Reduction of Adipose Tissue and Body Weight: Effect of Water-Soluble Calcium Hydroxycitrate in Garcinia Atroviridis on the Short-Term Treatment of Obese Women in Thailand." *Asia Pacific Journal of Clinical Nutrition* 16, no. 1 (2007): 25–29.

Schulze, M. B., M. Schulz, C. Heidemann, A. Schienkiewitz, K. Hoffmann, and H. Boeing. "Fiber and Magnesium Intake and Incidence of Type 2 Diabetes: A Prospective Study and Meta-analysis." *Archives of Internal Medicine* 167 (2007): 956–65.

Sethumadhavan, S., and P. Chinnakannu. "L-Carnitine and Alpha-Lipoic Acid Improve Age-Associated Decline in Mitochondrial Respiratory Chain Activity of Rat Heart Muscle." *Journals of Gerontology Series A: Biological Sciences and Medical Sciences* 61, no. 7 (2006): 650–59.

Volpe, S. L., H. W. Huang, K. Larpadisorn, and I. I. Lesser. "Effect of Chromium Supplementation and Exercise on Body Composition, Resting Metabolic Rate, and Selected Biochemical Parameters in Moderately Obese Women Following an Exercise Program." *Journal of the American College of Nutrition* 20, no. 4 (2001): 293–306.

Winkler, P., M. de Vrese, C. Laue, and J. H. Schrezenmeir. "Effect of a Dietary Supplement Containing Probiotic Bacteria plus Vitamins and Minerals on Common Cold Infections and Cellular Immune Parameters." *International Journal of Clinical Pharmacology and Therapeutics* 43, no. 7 (July 2005): 318–26.

Xu, J., X. F. Yang, H. L. Guo, X. H. Hou, L. G. Liu, and X. F. Sun. "Selenium Supplement Alleviated the Toxic Effects of Excessive Iodine in Mice." *Biological Trace Element Research* 111, no. 1–3 (Summer 2006): 229–38.

Zhang, H., K. Osada, H. Sone, and Y. Furukawa. "Biotin Administration Improves the Impaired Glucose Tolerance of Streptozotocin-Induced Diabetic Wistar Rats." *Journal of Nutritional Science and Vitaminology* 43, no. 3 (1997): 271–80.

Ziegler, D., A. Ametov, A. Barinov, P. J. Dyck, I. Gurieva, P. A. Low, U. Munzel, et al. "Oral Treatment with Lipoic Acid Improves Symptomatic Diabetic Polyneuropathy: The SYDNEY 2 Trial." *Diabetes Care* 29 (2006): 2365–70.

CHAPTER 10

Bent, S., A. Padula, D. Moore, M. Patterson, and W. Mehling. "Valerian for Sleep: A Systematic Review and Meta-analysis." *American Journal of Medicine* 119, no. 12 (December 2006): 1005–12.

Dallman, M. F., N. C. Pecoraro, and S. E. la Fleur. "Chronic Stress and Comfort Foods: Self-Medication and Abdominal Obesity." *Brain, Behavior, and Immunity* 19, no. 4 (July 2005): 275–80.

Kripke, D. F. "Greater Incidence of Depression with Hypnotic Use Than with Placebo." *BMC Psychiatry* 7: 42; doi: 10. 1186/1471-244X-7-42.

Maxwell, C., and S. L. Volpe. "Effect of Zinc Supplementation on Thyroid Hormone Function: A Case Study of Two College Females." *Annals of Nutrition and Metabolism* 51, no. 2 (2007): 188–94.

Steptoe, A., and J. Wardle. "Cardiovascular Stress Responsivity, Body Mass, and Abdominal Adiposity." *International Journal of Obesity* 29, no. 11 (November 2005): 1329–37.

CHAPTER 11

Ballor, D. L. "Effect of Dietary Restriction and/or Exercise on 23-Hour Metabolic Rate and Body Composition in Female Rats." *Journal of Applied Physiology* 71, no. 3 (September 1991): 801–806.

Ballor, D. L., and V. L. Katch. "Strength Gains in Obese Females Are Unaffected by Moderate Dietary Restriction." *European Journal of Applied Physiology and Occupational Physiology* 59, no. 5 (1989): 351–54.

Ballor, D. L., V. L. Katch, M. D. Becque, and C. R. Marks. "Resistance Weight Training during Caloric Restriction Enhances Lean Body Weight Maintenance." *American Journal of Clinical Nutrition* 47, no. 1 (January 1988): 19–25.

Hamer, M., and A. Steptoe. "Association between Physical Fitness, Parasympathetic Control, and Pro-inflammatory Responses to Mental Stress." *Psychosomatic Medicine* 69, no. 7 (August 2007): 660–666.

Kristal, A. R., A. J. Littman, D. Benitez, and E. White. "Yoga Practice Is Associated with Attenuated Weight Gain in Healthy, Middle-Aged Men and Women." *Alternative Therapies in Health and Medicine* 11, no. 4 (July-August 2005): 10–2, 28–33.

Redman, L., and E. Ravussin. "Effect of Calorie Restriction with or without Exercise on Body Composition and Fat Distribution." *Journal of Clinical Endocrinology & Metabolism* 92, no. 3 (March 2007): 865–872.

Shaibi, G. Q., M. L. Cruz, G. D. Ball, M. J. Weigensberg, G. J. Salem, N. C. Crespo, and M. I. Goran. "Effects of Resistance Training on Insulin Sensitivity in Overweight Latino Adolescent Males." *Medicine and Science in Sports and Exercise* 38, no. 7 (July 2006): 1208–15.

Westcott, W. L. "The Scoop on Super Slow Strength Training." *IDEA Personal Trainer* (November-December 1999): 37–42.

Westcott, W. L., R. A. Winett, E. S. Anderson, J. R. Wojcik, R. L. R. Loud, E. Cleggett, and S. Glover. "Effects of Regular and Slow Speed Resistance Training on Muscle Strength." *Journal of Sports Medicine and Physical Fitness* 41 (2001): 154–58.

CHAPTER 12

Moreno, J. A., F. Perez-Jimenez, C. Marin, P. Gomez, P. Perez-Martinez, R. Moreno, C. Bellido, F. Fuentes, and J. Lopez-Miranda. "The Effect of Dietary Fat on LDL Side Is Influenced by Apolipoprotein E Genotype in Healthy Subjects." *Journal of Nutrition* 134 (October 2004): 2517–22.

CHAPTER 14

Calles-Escandon, J., M. I. Goran, M. O'Connell, K. S. Nair, and E. Danforth. "Exercise Increases Fat Oxidation at Rest Unrelated to Changes in Energy Balance or Lipolysis." *American Journal of Physiology* 270, no. 6[1] (1996): e1009–14.

Jacobs, I., H. Lithell, and J. Karlsson. "Dietary Effects on Lipoprotein Lipase Activity in Skeletal Muscle in Man." *Acta Physiologica Scandinavica* 115 (1982): 85–90.

Lapachet, R. A. B., W. C. Miller, and D. A. Arnall. "Body Fat and Exercise Endurance in Trained Rats Adapted to a High-Fat and/or High-Carbohydrate Diet." *Journal of Applied Physiology* 80, no. 4 (1996): 1173–79.

Muio, D. M., J. J. Leddy, P. J. Horvath, A. B. Awad, and D. R. Pendergast. "Effect of Dietary Fat on Metabolic Adjustments to Maximal VO2 and Endurance in Runners." *Medicine and Science in Sports and Exercise* 26, no. 1 (1994): 81–88.

Phinney, S. D., B. R. Bistrian, W. J. Evans, E. Gervino, and G. I. Blackburn. "The Human Metabolic Response to Chronic Ketosis without Caloric Restriction: Preservation of Submaximal Exercise Capability with Reduced Carbohydrate Oxidation." *Metabolism* 32 (1983): 769–76.

INDEX

Boldface page references indicate references photographs. <u>Underscored</u> references indicate boxed text.

ABOUT THE AUTHORS

Keith Berkowitz, MD, is founder and medical director of the Center for Balanced Health in New York City and a former medical director of the Atkins Center for Complementary Medicine. He lives on Long Island, New York.

Valerie Berkowitz, MS, RD, is the director of nutrition at the Center for Balanced Health. Formerly a nutritionist at The Atkins Center, she serves as a nutrition consultant to *Prevention* and *Men's Health* magazines. She lives on Long Island, New York.

Alisa Bowman is a professional writer who has collaborated on more than 20 books, including 5 *New York Times* best-sellers. She lives in Emmaus, Pennsylvania with her husband, daughter, and dog.